The Last Diet

Cook Yourself Thin with Dr Eva

DR EVA ORSMOND MD MPH

GILL & MACMILLAN

Gill & Macmillan
Hume Avenue
Park West
Dublin 12
with associated companies throughout the world
www.gillmacmillan.ie

978 07171 5108 0

Design and print origination by www.grahamthew.com
Printed by GraphyCems, Spain

Index by Kate Murphy

The paper used in this book is made from the wood pulp of managed forests.
For every tree felled, at least one tree is planted, thereby renewing natural
resources.

PHOTO CREDITS
© Matteo Tuniz: front cover image, 10–11, 38–9, 44BL, 44TL, 52, 66, 81–3, 83
(inset), 102, 106, 109, 111, 112–13, 122, 125BM, 128, 138, 145, 146–7, 148, 150,
151, 155, 156–7, 161BL, 170, 182, 185, 19, 199, 211.

© Joanne Murphy: i, ii–iii, 2–3, 6–7, 23, 33, 44TR, 44MR, 44BR, 44ML, 47, 50,
55, 63, 65, 68, 69, 70, 89, 91, 93, 94, 97, 98, 100, 105, 125TL, 125TM, 125TR,
125BL, 125BR, 127, 130, 133, 135, 137, 140, 161TL, 161TR, 161ML, 161MR,
161FR, 161BM, 163, 164, 167, 169, 174, 177, 178, 181, 181, 189, 194–5, 203, 204,
206–207, 208, 209, 218; styled by Orla Neligan; assistant to photographer
and stylist: Carly Horan.

Props supplied by Avoca, Avoca Head Office, Kilmacanogue, Bray,
Co. Wicklow, T: 01 2746900, E: info@avoca.ie; Eden Home & Garden,
1–4 Temple Grove, Temple Road, Blackrock, Co. Dublin, T: 0 1 7642004,
W: www.edenhomeandgarden.ie; Meadows & Byrne, The Pavilion,
Royal Marine Road, Dun Laoghaire, Co. Dublin, T: 01 2804554,
W: www.meadowsandbyrne.com; Article, Powerscourt Townhouse, South
William Street, Dublin 2, T: 01 6799268, E: items@articledublin.com,
W: www.articledublin.com; Elizabelle, 23 Church Street, Listowel, Co. Kerry,
T: 068 22593, W: www.elizabelle.com. Other props by Ittala, Arabia and
Hackman. Eva's apron by Marimekko, W: www.marimekko.com.

Contents

List of recipes

Acknowledgments

This book would never have seen the daylight without the constant support, push and dedication that my husband Wyatt has always given to me. English is not my mother tongue and Wyatt has not only put the text in its readable version but also used his engineering logic to arrange things in some sensible order. Anybody who knows me knows that this book has been a long labour of love that started almost 10 years ago— only a few years after I had opened my first private weight-loss clinic. Holding the final printed version of my book in my hand is on the list of the highlights of my life after my wedding day and the births of my boys, and I am sure anybody who has written a book would agree and would say the same!

I would like to thank the many people in RTÉ who have encouraged and acknowledged my hard work and ambition by regularly inviting me to different radio and TV shows and interviews. I can mention only a few as the list is otherwise too long. Marty Whelan was my 'first' live interview on RTÉ's 'Open House' back in 2001! From that followed many interviews, radio and TV programmes with the highlight being 'The Late Late Show' with Pat Kenny! I was so nervous I did not sleep well a full week before the show where I presented 'The worst food for 2006'. Pat was a bit concerned when I arrived for rehearsal with my curlers on and just checked with me that I was going to take them off before the live show! Not only did I tick the box by having been on 'The Late Late Show', it also paved the way to being discovered by another 'important man' in my life— Philip Kampf of VIP Productions. Since then, things have just got better. Ireland and the Irish have been good to me and my family. The craic and love for life makes the Irish so special but this also often makes them unhealthy!

Even though I love my native country, Finland, and I am proud of my roots, I have found a place here and would like to call Ireland home. Thanks to everyone in my local community and former and present colleagues and hospital staff, who have given me such support. Please adopt me and try to understand that even though I am sometimes harsh and very direct, TOUGH LOVE is needed at times!

I want to thank all my staff at my clinics, especially Marie for being the 'second' me, keeping me organised and making sure everything runs when I am too busy! Katri, another Finn, who has stuck it out with me for so many years and who keeps striving to develop and learn more; Yvonne—the rock of the temple; Rachel—a ball of energy; and Michelle for all the help in analysing the recipes using WISP and for keeping track of the millions of changes. I would also like to thank the many patients I have met over the years—I have been lucky to meet so many people who have inspired and helped me.

To the staff at G&M, and particularly to Tess for the hard and very time-consuming editing task, thank you for your endless patience and attention to detail. Books like this don't see print without attention to detail, total dedication and deadlines. I love attention to detail!!!!

Thank You—*Kiitos!*

Eva

Introduction

In my mother's kitchen it used to be either a feast or a famine. Her homemade food was tasty but full of calories, and when we ate, we ate well. But her weight and mine would slowly creep up and then reality would strike and it was diet time. We would try all sorts of diets with a reward in mind. Once we got it, for example a holiday, it was soon back to old habits and the kilos piled on. So, by the time I had finished my schooling and medical degree, a constant awareness of body weight and the effects of different foods and diets was 'in my genes'. A few years later, while completing my Master's Degree in Public Health, obesity was being highlighted as a 'new epidemic' and the experts were all trying to find a solution to the increasing obesity levels. Even though the solution could be so simple—eat less and exercise more—in reality we all know it is not that easy!

With so much confusing advice out there and with all of us trying to find a quick way to lose weight, we are getting nowhere! I am not offering an easy way out, but we all need a little help. With simple weight-loss steps and tasty recipes, this book gives you the knowledge to help you achieve a healthy weight, in the same way patients in my clinics have done over the past 10 years.

My recipes and menus are a fusion of my Finnish roots and my mother's kitchen, my university years in Italy and my housewife childbearing years in South Africa. All these were combined with my new life in Ireland and attempts to maintain a healthy diet for myself, my two boys and husband. A never-ending challenge!

 I have managed to do it, my patients have managed to do it and now I will show you how you can do it too without being a master chef!

PS. Thirteen has always been my lucky number, so this book has 13 chapters.

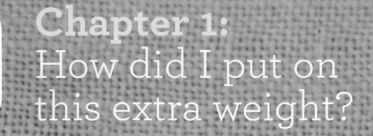

CHAPTER 1

Chapter 1:
How did I put on
this extra weight?

IN ORDER TO lose extra weight we have to look back and start figuring out when we started slowly, or quickly, piling on the pounds. Usually we can recall an event or period when this happened but in some cases obesity dates back to early childhood. History is important so that we can look back and correct what went wrong.

Obviously our sedentary lifestyle, with more people using cars and less physical activity, has an impact on our overall energy expenditure. We drive our children to school and would not dream of doing otherwise, but in our childhood we walked or cycled to school. The reasons for this are numerous but generally safety is the main issue. Things need to happen for us instantaneously these days and for this same reason we don't even want to spend time preparing a meal. Everything in our current lifestyle is geared to make us use less of our energy and use more fuel or other environmental energy, thus creating larger carbon footprints. Computer games are about as close to sport as some children get and watching TV is probably the most common childhood pastime. Not only are our children less active but they are also becoming less resourceful when it comes to childhood games because they are so used to passive entertainment. Although it is clear these environmental factors have reduced our physical activity and have contributed to our increasing weight, it is only a small part of the problem compared with the increased calorie intake in our everyday diet.

Then there are the most common day-to-day reasons for weight gain. The following are all contributory factors for increasing weight:

- Getting married
- Giving up smoking
- Becoming pregnant
- Changing jobs
- Going on holidays
- Going through puberty
- Going through menopause

- Moving to another country
- Starting to study
- Starting working, stopping working or retiring
- Giving up exercise or being less active
- Suffering from any form of serious illness
- Ageing
- Medical reasons (e.g. under-active thyroid, arthritis)
- Medication

All of the above have something in common—a change in routine.

We all have a routine that we follow. Even the most disorganised people have a 'no-routine', which is always the same. I have witnessed this very clearly in my clinic. Any change in routine inevitably changes what we eat and how many calories we burn. If this change causes an imbalance, it will affect our bodies either negatively or positively.

Weight gain is a very common and serious side effect of many commonly used drugs, for example antipsychotics, antidepressants, anti-convulsants (for epilepsy), anti-diabetic medications (insulin, and oral hypoglycaemic medication), steroids, beta blockers (very commonly used in the treatment of cardiovascular disease), etc. For some of these drugs the mechanism of action is fairly well understood, but for many others this remains unknown. If any of these drugs causes weight gain, they should be reviewed as alternatives are available.

Regardless of who you are or what your history is, if you eat (take in energy) in excess of what your body requires, then your body will store this energy as fat. There is no escape from this. As we are all unique, every individual has different energy needs and energy consumption. Even if you have a tendency to put on weight, it does not mean that you will inevitably gain weight. The fact is that on average we put on 0.5–2kg (1.1–4.4 lb) every year unless it is actively managed. Consider the following: one biscuit has about 75 calories—if you ate 75 calories more than your body needed every day, over a period of one month this could result in approximately 300 g of extra weight, eventually leading to as much as 3.6 kg (half a stone) a year.

Taking into account all the additional health risks you are exposing yourself to, it's no wonder that obesity is considered a chronic disease. Aside from the obvious physical health risks, I consider the silent negative psychological impact especially damaging.

Your everyday quality of life is diminished not only by the burden of carrying all that extra weight, but every moment of the day you are reminded that you are too 'big'.

You find that you can't do things you used to do such as tie your shoelaces, clothes don't fit, the tummy love handles become a spare tyre, you puff around the golf course and by the evening, when you finally have time for yourself, you fall asleep in front of the TV, exhausted. I could carry on and on as the list of disadvantages is endless, but then again so are the positive benefits of weight reduction.

The traditional nutritional guidelines are not helping either. The disparity between what is right and what is wrong is huge. There are 'eat fat and get slim' and 'low fat high carb' diets that many of us have tried with varied success. I do not consider either to be the right way—nothing will work as well as a balanced diet. We are given different and contradictory messages all the time about food and how to lose weight. So, how do you know that the message I am giving is the right one? I suppose you have to ask yourself if what I say makes sense, then it's up to you to put it into practice. When you see how your health and your frame of mind improves as the excess weight slowly leaves you, you should be convinced. If you follow my advice, this time you won't see the excess weight returning—it will be gone forever.

In nutrition there are a few rules that you can't change and these are:

- Calories count—energy can neither be created nor destroyed (1st law of thermodynamics).
- Our body reacts differently to different foods (this is explained in Chapter 3 under 'Glycaemic Index').
- A continued negative energy balance will create weight loss.
- Our body needs a combination of macronutrients (protein, fat and carbohydrates) and micronutrients (vitamins and minerals) to function optimally. In other words, we need a balanced diet.
- Excessive weight loss or excessive weight gain can both conceivably lead to death.

First, we need to stop fooling ourselves and admit that food plays a huge role in our lives.

BABIES ARE NOT BORN FAT!

My first baby was born in Finland in 1996 while it was -22 °C outside. Being a Finn and a doctor meant I knew what was best and breastfeeding was obviously going to give my child the best start. All scientific data has proven that breastfeeding reduces and prevents allergic conditions. As I had allergies, I was going to prevent this happening to my child! Things didn't start smoothly as I wasn't producing enough milk so I ended up feeding the baby every two hours and I was exhausted.

A few months later my baby became uncomfortable and we ended up at a paediatrician. This middle-aged but experienced man reassured us that our child was fine but immediately told me that he was overweight. This was the last thing I would have ever expected to hear. He asked about our routine. What routine? The baby ate and slept as it came naturally and I did my utmost to cater to his every need.

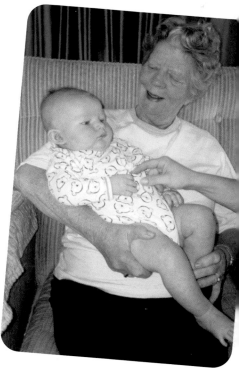

The doctor sent us to a nurse who set a new feeding routine that included small amounts of solids with the promise that in two weeks' time the child would sleep through the night and give me back some of my life. Vegetables were mashed and introduced to the child slowly to get his taste and gastric system used to new flavours and consistencies of foods. His feeding intervals were set like clockwork and we were to follow the routine with German precision. Anyway, it worked. In less than two weeks our baby was sleeping through the night and had become a lot more settled.

This is my experience but you need to treat each child's case individually, and if you can't breastfeed, it's not the end of the world. I know this is not a book about bringing up children and everyone has their own thoughts on this matter (I am no expert), but what this did teach me was how important diet is from the start of our lives.

Obviously an essential part of this new routine was the fact that the child was not hungry and his needs were satisfied. By my baby's first birthday he was well in line with growth charts and the excess weight had disappeared. I was cooking all his meals from scratch and he was getting balanced and tasty food. Every new taste was a new experience. Sometimes he accepted it with delight, but sometimes it required some convincing and perseverance.

If I had not met this upfront doctor and wise nurse my baby could have grown to childhood overweight, possibly obese, with the potential to develop a huge number of food dislikes.

Even when the consequences of being overweight or obese are highlighted to the general public, parents still tend to be in denial over their own children. They want to believe that it is just puppy fat and will disappear on its own. Unfortunately, about 70 per cent of overweight children will eventually become obese adults, developing Type 2 diabetes, heart disease, high blood pressure and even some forms of cancer. These chronically ill young adults will not be able to enjoy their youth because of their parents' lack of willpower to say no to their children's demands for fast food, fizzy drinks and big portions.

Your example is the most powerful. If you change, they will follow.

Chapter 2:
Calories count

THERE ARE SOME lucky people who don't have to count their money but everybody has to count their calories. Yes, initially you will need to actually count them and keep control of your intake, but with time you will learn to understand food and the whole process becomes as natural as being aware of your bank balance.

What are calories? Calories are the energy found in food. One kilo-calorie (kcal) is equivalent to the energy needed to increase the temperature of a gram of water by 1 °C.

You will always find some new diet that claims that you can eat as much as you want of certain foods, but, in reality, calories are the energy that your body uses and if you give it too much it gets stored as fat. Think about it this way—fuel is the energy your car uses, and you keep it in balance by filling it up when necessary. If you put too much fuel in, it overflows. This would be seen as a stupid mistake, so why do we do it to our bodies? Unfortunately, your body cannot overflow but stores the excess energy as fat and will carry on doing so. The bottom line is that calories count.

If you want to use up the excess stored energy, you have to put less energy (food) into your body than it needs so that it will burn your reserves. This energy will come from fat and lean muscular mass. By selecting the foods correctly, you can minimise the lean muscular mass loss and maximise the use of the fat reserves.

> **IN ORDER TO LOSE WEIGHT YOU NEED TO CREATE A NEGATIVE ENERGY BALANCE.**

In brief, current guidelines recommend that an average adult woman can eat approximately 2,000 kcal per day to maintain her weight and an average adult man can eat approximately 2,500 kcal per day to maintain his weight.

There are various methods to calculate your daily average calorie consumption. They take into account height, weight, activity levels, age and gender. They will give you an indication of calorie consumption but cannot be considered accurate.

The best way is to work out your own calorie consumption by keeping an accurate diet diary for 1 week. It's a bit laborious but it's the most accurate way.

To lose weight, you need to consume fewer calories than you require so that the body will be forced to use your stored fat as energy. Unfortunately, if you reduce your food intake by only a small amount, you are not going to achieve anything as we tend to underestimate the amount of food we consume daily and are likely to forget about that quick snack or glass of juice. To initially lose weight effectively, a significant drop in calorie intake over an extended period is required. For example, a 7,500 kcal energy deficit will result in 1 kg (2.2 lb) weight loss. It is important to note that when you lose weight, your daily calorie requirement will also reduce. This is why some people hit a 'plateau' in their weight-loss attempts. This means that you will need to reduce your calorie intake further to achieve continued weight loss.

Body Mass Index (BMI)

Do you know your present weight? You might think you do but it could be that the number you have in mind is actually a number that you remember from six months ago or longer. We are getting heavier every day so if you think you are heavy now, you are probably still lighter than you will be in six months' time. That's if you don't actively do something about it now!

Let's start with a basic assessment. The currently accepted way of assessing your fat status is by calculating your BMI or Body Mass Index. In simple terms, BMI is an indication of the amount of weight you carry per square metre of skin.

HOW TO CALCULATE YOUR BMI

To calculate your BMI, all you need is a good, accurate—preferably digital—weighing scales, a metric tape measure and a calculator. First, weigh yourself in kilograms. Next measure your height in metres as accurately as possible. (Do not rely on measurements you remember from a few months or years ago.) Now divide your weight (in kg) by your height (in m) squared as follows:

$$\frac{\text{WEIGHT (KG)}}{\text{HEIGHT x HEIGHT (M)}} = \text{BMI (kg/m}^2)$$

If your BMI is:

<18.5—you are underweight

18.5 to 24.9—you are in the normal weight range

25 to 29.9—you are overweight

>30—you are obese—Class I

>35—Class II obese

>40—Class III morbidly obese

A BMI over 40 is Class III and regarded as morbidly obese because your health is severely at risk. The BMI cut-off ranges are indicative of the effect that body weight has on disease and death. The higher the BMI, the greater the risk of developing certain conditions, including diabetes, high cholesterol, heart disease, particular cancers, and the obvious wear and tear on the joints due to the weight. Alternatively, the lower the BMI, the greater the risk of malnutrition and osteoporosis.

BMI is a useful indicator but it is not 100 per cent reliable. For instance, age is a factor. BMI ranges are based on population ages of 18–65 years old and so it is not suitable for people who are younger or older. In South East Asia, the BMI ranges are also slightly different. Another disadvantage of BMI is that it does not take into account body composition. In this way it might class someone who has a very high muscle mass as obese even though they are a perfectly normal weight. This is because muscle is heavier in volume than fat and therefore increases the weight of a lean body. BMI can also underestimate the degree of obesity in individuals, particularly the elderly, who have a very low muscle mass. For this reason observation plays a key role in conjunction with BMI to assess whether the results seem realistic.

BMI was first used by insurance companies to calculate quotes for life insurance taken out after the Second World War and it was based on mortality statistics. The insurance industry long ago recognised that men and women taking out insurance policies were likely to die early if they were overweight, especially if they were obese when young. People's insurance rates were based on their weight and consequently risk of disease amongst other things. Even today it is still used when assessing life insurance.

If the number you got from your calculation is a BMI >30, you are obese. It is only a word but this word means that you are suffering from a chronic disease and that at some stage you will suffer from its physical consequences. If you are overweight, instead of obese, your risks are lower but there is still work to do. Remember, all obese people were once overweight.

Healthy weight should not be seen as a number but rather a range within which your weight does not increase your health risks. For example, a person whose height is 1.63 m (approximately 5 ft 4 inches) will have a healthy weight of between 50 kg (7 st 12 lb) and 66 kg (10 st 5 lb) or in BMI terms 18.5 to 24.9. However, a BMI of 24.9 is verging on overweight and so the ideal BMI is about 21 to 22—in this case 56 to 59 kg (8 st 11 lb to 9 st 4 lb).

At my clinic when I ask people during their first assessment what their current weight is, most of them don't even know it. Many come to see me thinking that they are overweight and need to lose a few pounds, but in most cases they are in fact clinically obese. I remember a particular lady who was so shocked when she heard that she was obese, she carried on repeating it every time I saw her.

However, she managed to lose the weight very quickly and maintained her new weight as well. So, if you are overweight or obese, face the facts and start doing something about it now!

OTHER FAT MEASUREMENTS

There are other ways to measure your fat status such as fat percentage through electrical scales that you can buy in pharmacies, but these are not accurate. However, the waistline measurement is the most important.

If you are overweight, it is important to know where that excess fat is located. Is it around your hips or around your waist? This is where the waist measurement is important because it indicates the presence of central obesity. Despite its simplicity, waist circumference has been shown to be an accurate predictor of intra-abdominal fat, either alone or in combination with BMI. Having a large waist circumference (apple shape) indicates increased risk to health compared with peripheral obesity, i.e. weight on the hips or being 'pear shaped'. Abdominal fat is an independent risk factor for disease for those with a BMI within the healthy weight range. What this means is that medical research is now convinced that visceral fat that accumulates around your waist is very dangerous and increases your risk of different diseases. The main ones are diabetes and high cholesterol, which lead to heart disease. For older people and those from different ethnic backgrounds, waist circumference is a better indicator of health than BMI.

The waist circumference is measured just above the belly button. It is important to ensure that the tape is snug but not tight and that you are not breathing in.

Waist measurements as a predictor of risk to health
(World Health Organization, 2000)

	Increased risk	Substantial risk
Caucasian men	>94 cm (37 inches)	>102 cm (40 inches)
Caucasian women	>80 cm (32 inches)	>88 cm (35 inches)
Asian men	No data	>90 cm (36 inches)
Asian women	No data	>80 cm (32 inches)

Note: waist measurements are taken at the navel.

Each 1 kg (2.2 lb) of weight loss should drop your waist measurement by 1 cm.

Chapter 3:
What on earth are you eating!

SIXTY PER CENT of adults and 20 per cent of children and teens in Ireland are classified as overweight or obese and we are currently the second fattest nation in Europe. However, studies have found that the Irish are not alone—since the sixties, in the United States, the level of overweight/obesity has risen to 1 in 4 children and 1 in 2 adults.

Over the past 10 years we have gone through the information era. We have instant access to almost any information via the internet, and are kept up to date with international news and the latest health scares (SARS, Avian Flu). However, when it comes to eating and diet, we have faltered. Fast food and fizzy drinks are now considered acceptable elements of a normal diet and vegetables and fruit are seen as old-fashioned. There no longer appears to be time for proper home cooking. So what has gone wrong? Is our education on food that poor?

Most of us have seen the classic food pyramid either in a classroom, doctor's surgery, local chemist or at the supermarket. Although you may not have taken much notice of it or tried to do what it suggests, the pyramid depicts the hierarchy of food types and their importance in the diet.

The base of the pyramid contains starchy bread, potatoes, rice and cereal, and fat, oil, butter and sweets form the peak. The layout emphasises the importance of low fat and recommends complex carbohydrates as the main source of our daily energy. This pyramid was conceived in the USA in the 1960s as a result of an increase in cardiovascular disease. The graphic representation of the Food Guide Pyramid was released only in 1992 to promote healthy eating. However, it does not appear to be working because the countries advocating it are all getting fatter.

So what's the problem with this food pyramid? In my opinion, it's the bottom level—too much carbohydrate and no separation between 'good' and 'bad' carbohydrates. I don't think that bread and potatoes should form the foundation of a meal. Think of a typical takeaway meal, e.g. hamburger and chips—it's basically bread and potatoes. Is this a healthy meal even if you add a few pieces of tomato and have a glass of milk with it? Of course not, but more shockingly, neither is a bowl of processed cereal.

The next problem with the pyramid is the ambiguity of portion size and the calories associated with different food types. Even by taking typical serving volumes and food preferences, the food pyramid is suitable only for an active man of normal weight who does not drink alcohol.

We have become obsessed with eating but complacent about food choice. Eating out or getting a takeaway are now everyday events not a special treat. It's easier and almost cheaper to buy readymade meals than cooking at home. We don't really know what we are eating and wouldn't have the knowledge to judge even if we were informed. The takeaway industry has thrived on our ignorance and modern fast-paced lifestyle and, being profit-based, uses the most cost-effective methods and ingredients to make its products. These include taste enhancers, preservatives and bulking agents to mention a few. The concept of a balanced meal has fallen by the wayside.

Even the medical profession often fails to acknowledge the importance of diet as a cause of disease and illness. When we go and see the doctor due to ill health, they seldom ask us about our diet. It's quicker and easier to simply prescribe medication to alleviate a symptom. Take the common complaint of constipation—doctors simply give the patient a laxative and advise them to increase fibre intake. Why are you constipated in the first place? Well, take a good look at your diet—where are the vegetables, the fruit, etc.? Is your diet balanced?

When you go to the supermarket, what jumps out at you and what are you selecting? Is it the added vitamins or 'diet option'? How about 'no added sugar' or, my personal favourite 'low fat'? I am not knocking these products but there is a difference in quality between all the products. Please do not be under the impression that one product will change your life!

The Glycaemic Index (GI)

The Glycaemic Index (GI) was originally developed in 1981 as a better way to classify carbohydrates than referring to them as 'simple' or 'complex'. Nowadays it is used more extensively and most common foods have been given a GI ranking.

The Glycaemic Index is a way of evaluating and ranking foods according to how quickly they increase blood sugar levels when eaten. Foods with a high GI enter the bloodstream rapidly, while low glycaemic foods promote a slower release of glucose (blood sugar) into the bloodstream.

When glucose enters the bloodstream, it increases blood sugar levels. This increase causes the pancreas to release insulin, a hormone that activates cells to absorb the glucose. If we get a rapid increase in glucose absorption—hence rapidly increasing blood sugar levels—we get a compensatory rapid increase in insulin. Because our body does not need all this energy (glucose) immediately, the insulin signals the body to store away the energy for later use—usually as fat. This storage process happens rapidly (due to the high insulin levels), and the body experiences a rapid drop in blood sugar levels. This sends a signal to the brain that it needs food again.

However, if we eat food that is not absorbed rapidly into the blood and does not cause blood sugar levels to rise rapidly, only a minimal amount of insulin is released and the glucose is used up as energy and not stored. As the use of this energy is gradual and lasting, the blood sugar levels tend to stay level for longer and so do the insulin levels. The effect of this is that we start receiving signals that we need more energy only when it is actually required. These foods are called low glycaemic foods.

For practical purposes foods are classified into low (below 55), medium (55–70) and high GI (above 70) based on their GI ranking from 0 to 100.

HOW IS THE GLYCAEMIC INDEX OF FOOD ESTABLISHED?

A test subject is given a 50 g portion of glucose (called the control portion) and their blood sugar levels are monitored. They are then given a portion of test food and their blood sugar levels are again monitored. The test food is given an index based on these results.

White bread can also be used as the control portion. It has a Glycaemic Index about 35 points lower than glucose. To be specific, this bread is called white wheat bread (WWB). So when you are looking at a table showing the GI of foods, make sure you know what it is based on, either glucose or WWB. I suggest you use the tables with glucose as the base because they are less confusing.

Unfortunately, the glycaemic indexing of food is not an exact science and there are a number of factors that can significantly change the Index. Some of these are:

- **Type of carbohydrate, fibre content, macro- and micro-nutrient content**
- **Types of preservatives used**
- **Method of food processing and cooking**
- **Ripeness of food and food storage methods**

Furthermore, as we are all different and our body's response to food varies, the GI will also change. So, we need to be careful not to be too specific about the GI of a food but to rather look at it in general. In essence, foods that have a GI of less than 50 are low glycaemic and should make up most of your diet.

The Food and Agriculture Organization of the United Nations (FAO) and WHO endorse the use of the GI. However, despite the evidence, the use of the GI has not reached a universal consensus. The main criticism is due to the fact that foods are usually eaten in combination, i.e. bread is normally eaten with butter, and this lowers the GI of the bread. There are some anomalies too, such as peanuts and chocolate having a low GI, whereas a baked potato has a high GI.

This is the main reason why we need to look at the bigger picture and don't concentrate only on one factor in our diet. Calories still count.

I don't want you to be obsessed by the GI value only. For example, a large salad of lettuce, cucumber and mushrooms will have a very low GI and will have hardly any calories but it also has hardly any fibre, which means you will still be feeling very hungry half an hour or so later. So how does this help you? If used correctly, the low glycaemic diet will allow us to eat larger quantities that will keep us satisfied for longer. Certain foods (like dark chocolate) have a lower GI than watermelon. How could you possibly lose weight eating plenty of dark chocolate instead of watermelon?

Food dislikes

Take a minute and write down which foods you don't like and which you would not eat under any circumstances. If the list is long, then you are in trouble!

Having food dislikes is a common occurrence today. Adults now have many food dislikes but our young people have even more. It's shocking to say that if we do not change this soon, in 20 years' time vegetable agriculture may not even exist. The most commonly eaten and liked vegetables are peas, corn and carrots. Vegetables such as broccoli, cabbage, cauliflower, courgette, aubergine, fennel and butternut are less popular. Some young people have never even tasted vegetables as common as cucumber and pepper.

Limited diet choices, especially in the vegetable group, make it impossible to create an appetising and interesting diet that fills you up and gives you all the fibre, vitamins and minerals your body needs. Usually people who have a long list of food dislikes prefer bread and sweet things and this is one of the biggest reasons for their weight gain. You can grow out of sweet cravings and that overwhelming need to eat all the time, but in order to succeed you must have a balanced diet that feeds your body's nutritional needs.

Food dislikes are a bad thing and one of the biggest obstacles to weight reduction—but this can change if you want it to.

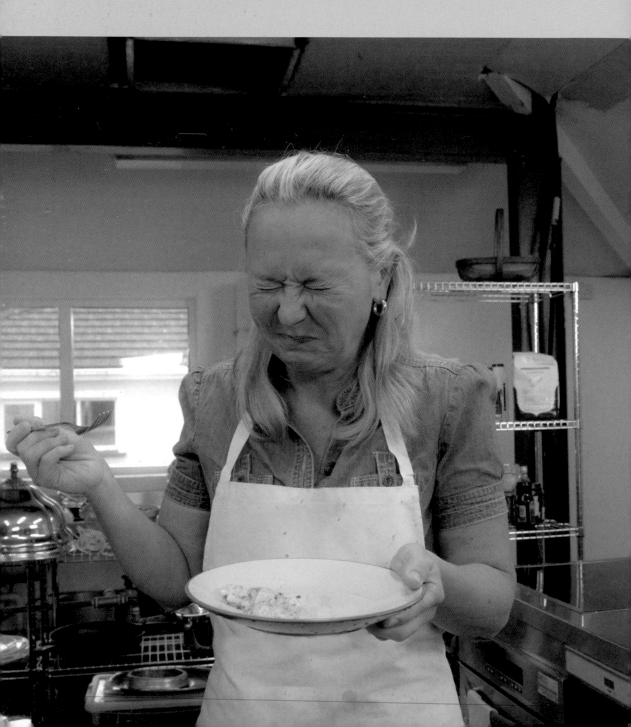

Diets—good and bad

There are numerous diets available today—the Atkins Diet, Cabbage Soup Diet, Montignac Method, Nutron Diet, South Beach Diet, the Dukan Diet, System 10, Zone Diet—as well as food replacements such as protein bars, drinks, many supplements like apple vinegar extract tablets. There are also fat-absorbing tablets, fat-melting pants, vibrating belts and hundreds of diet books. Added to this you have light crisps, low fat yoghurts, low fat bread, low fat everything. Every possible 'easy' solution seems to be out there but yet we continue to get heavier.

I have often been asked if this or that diet is unhealthy or maybe even dangerous to our health. My answer is simple—the diet is probably not going to kill you but the weight might. Generally, nobody can follow an unnatural diet regime for long enough to create permanent damage to their health. Furthermore, once they stop following the diet, it doesn't take long for them to return to their old eating habits—and all the weight they lost, and more, comes back.

One positive element of faddy diets is that when you start losing weight quickly, you get motivated by the immediate weight loss. However, the reality is that even if the weight initially drops quickly, this does not carry on for very long and the lack of continued rapid success makes most people give up.

So, other than frustration, why don't these faddy diets work in the long term? Simple:

- **They don't create a lifestyle change that is based on a healthy eating routine.**
- **They are not flexible enough to be followed in life's different situations.**
- **They are unbalanced and unrealistic.**
- **They do not educate the dieter about food and food choices.**

There is a common belief that the slower you lose the weight, the more likely you are to keep it off. This is something I strongly believe in. If you lose the weight slowly, you are more likely to incorporate the change in diet into a 'new' lifestyle and maintain your weight loss. However, from a psychological point of view, rapid initial weight loss is more motivating, but the diet must then evolve into a slower, sustainable regime.

Different types of diets

VLC DIETS
Very Low Calorie Diets, or VLCDs, as the name suggests, are diets that use specifically formulated products that have a very low calorie content. However, if formulated correctly, the products still have all the other nutrients (proteins, vitamins and minerals) that the body needs. A VLCD is only a method of

reducing the weight, not a method of weight maintenance or weight management. Long-term results are achievable only if, after the diet, eating behaviour and activity levels are changed.

These diets are usually based on a 600–800 kcal daily intake and have been used with good results in recognised obesity clinics and hospitals. I use them in my clinics in certain circumstances. The idea is based on a high protein low carbohydrate diet where your body goes into ketosis, a state in which the body's fat is burned for energy, and this suppresses the appetite. The diet incorporates a large amount of vegetables with low carbohydrate content.

The diet is supplemented with products of high protein content with high biological value that contain all the vitamins and minerals needed by the body but very low in carbohydrates. These products are generally in powder form. When mixed with cold or hot water, they become soups or different types of creamy desserts like chocolate mousse. Alternatively, they are produced as snack bars.

A five-year follow up study showed good long-term results for those people able to stick to the diet long enough to achieve significant weight loss. The reason why this type of dramatic weight loss works so well is that it is based on the great motivation that people experience when they feel the benefits of weight loss after a relatively short period of time. Owing to the rapid weight loss and ketone state, it is important that your basic metabolic functions are normal and it is recommended that these diets are done under medical supervision.

PER CENT-SPECIFIC DIETS
These diets advocate eating specific percentages of carbohydrates, fats and proteins in every meal or snack in order to maintain the appropriate 'insulin zone'. A typical example would be a ratio of exactly 40 per cent carbohydrates, 30 per cent fat and 30 per cent protein. These diets generally recommend less than 800 kcal energy intake. These Very Low Calorie Diets should be medically supervised. My opinion is that it is very difficult to maintain such an exact intake of protein, carbohydrates and fat in every meal. This is not a perfect world and our lives are full of unexpected situations.

BLOOD-TYPE BASED
An 'Eat right for your blood type diet' is based on the principle that different people have different blood types and that only certain foods go well with certain blood types. For example, those with blood type A should avoid aubergines, cabbage, mushrooms and tomatoes—just to mention a few. These typical Mediterranean vegetables are very healthy and are actually the ones I usually recommend because they are low in calories, are low glycaemic and have been considered to be 'anti-cancer vegetables'. It is difficult to believe the theory behind this diet but for some it seems to work. There is not enough scientific evidence for this and more research is needed.

Another one of these blood-based diets determines an individual's tolerance or intolerance to 92 commonly consumed foods. Apparently by eliminating foods on the 'intolerant list', an individual can lose weight and gain energy. Again, this is unbalanced, excludes whole food groups and provides little food education.

LOW GI (NO CALORIE COUNTING)
There are diets that are based on the low glycaemic concept but they still have their shortfalls. Some undervalue the importance of calories and the quantities that can be consumed. Nuts, for example, are low glycaemic and very healthy because their oils are mainly polyunsaturated but they are very rich in calories.

FOOD REPLACEMENT DIETS
A portion or all of a meal is replaced by a product, typically a shake or a bar. The idea behind this diet is that the replacement meal has fewer calories than an ordinary meal. It makes a diet simple, as people don't usually have the knowledge to create low calorie meals. By sticking to the diet, your calorie intake is less than what your body burns and you will lose weight. However, if you eat too many calories during your allowed 'ordinary food', you might still not lose weight. These replacement meals are generally nutritionally balanced but they don't create any understanding of why you put the weight on in the first place and how to keep it off in the long term. The difference between these food replacement diets and VLCDs is that they don't reduce your appetite and can also lack sufficient fibre.

HIGH PROTEIN AND FAT, LOW CARBOHYDRATE DIET
This diet is based on unlimited protein and fat intake. All carbohydrates, like bread, potatoes and even fruit, have to be excluded. This diet can give quick and substantial initial weight loss based on the fact that proteins have a good satiating effect and you feel fuller for longer. The appetite is also suppressed by the ketone bodies that derive from fat. Anybody with heart or kidney function problems could run a health risk created by the electrolyte disturbances that can result from this diet. Some people find this diet appealing because of the unlimited meat and fat intake, which makes this diet sound so very easy to follow. The long-term effects on health from the unlimited consumption of saturated fats have been proven to be detrimental.

CABBAGE SOUP DIET
This diet is based on having as much cabbage soup as you want for breakfast, lunch and dinner. After a few days you are allowed a few extra items, for example fruit. Cabbage is very low in calories and if you burn more calories than you take in, you will obviously lose weight. Some people complain that this soup creates a lot of gas.

Any diet that is based on 1 to 2 food groups to the exclusion of others is unbalanced and cannot be good for you in the long term. It is unlikely that after a diet like this you will be able to maintain your weight loss because you will not have learned about portion control or gained any knowledge about nutrition and the other foods that make you gain weight.

Misleading labels and deceiving advertising

THE PRINCIPAL FUNCTION OF FOOD LABELLING IS TO INFORM CONSUMERS OF THE PROPERTIES OF PRE-PACKAGED FOOD. THE FUNDAMENTAL RULE OF THE LABELLING OF FOODSTUFFS IS THAT CONSUMERS SHOULD NOT BE MISLED. DETAILED LABELLING OF A PRODUCT EDUCATES CONSUMERS AS TO THE EXACT NATURE AND CHARACTER-ISTICS OF THE FOODSTUFF AND ENABLES THEM TO MAKE A MORE INFORMED CHOICE.

'Understanding Food Labelling', The Food Safety Authority of Ireland

The message of this leaflet is simple—educate yourself and don't be misled.

The larger more reputable companies would not usually mislead or have incorrect labelling as they know that it could risk their brand trust. However, some of them do know how to play the marketing game to their advantage because they know the law and how to advertise. For example, if you think a processed breakfast cereal is a healthy option, then you should have a good look at what nutritional value is contained in the bowl you are about to eat.

Another cereal-related misconception is the nutritional value per serving or per portion. The nutritional information is also given when served with skimmed-milk, so where is the nutrition actually coming from, the cereal or the milk?

How can simply having a small pot of yoghurt with some added vitamins and probiotics magically improve your health? Well, it can't. It is better than nothing but a balanced diet will give you all the nutrition and vitamins you need—plus more.

A very good example of how these companies use the lay person's nutritional ignorance to their advantage is outlined on p.119 in relation to fibre content.

I could carry on and on but the simple point is this—don't be misled and keep an open mind.

READING FOOD LABELS

It would be great if our daily diet could consist of foods that have been prepared fresh from basic ingredients by ourselves rather than pre-packed processed food. In reality we are just too busy and have other things to do, 'forcing' us to eat a certain amount of processed foods. However, this is not an excuse to forget about nutrition. There can be some major differences between food products and it is therefore important that we know how to read the labels. This will help you choose the 'real' healthier product with the best overall value, not simply the cheapest product with the loudest claims. The product we bought last time that tasted good will tempt us, but what is behind that good taste?

There are a few basics to food labelling. The rules and regulations do vary between countries but in general they are very similar.

The Product Name: This cannot be misleading. If it says it contains something, it must be true. There are some names that are 'legal' and these relate to specific products, e.g. milk chocolate must have >25 per cent cocoa solids.

List of Ingredients: All the ingredients must be listed and in descending order of weight. This is not compulsory for fresh fruit and vegetables or for products where the trade name is the same as the ingredient name, e.g. pepper.

Nutritional Information: Although this information is required by law only when a nutritional claim is made on the label, many manufacturers are now adding nutritional information to all their products. The nutrient values must be stated per 100 g or 100 ml and the energy levels given in kilojoules (kJ) or kilocalories (kcal).

Other: The product should be date-marked and state its weight and the manufacturer's name—this all helps to confirm its quality.

A lot of this information can be confusing or misleading. Claims like 'low fat', 'no added sugar', 'gluten free', 'high fibre', etc. need to be backed up and this is done using the nutritional information.

When looking at the calories, be careful that you are considering the package size. In some cases the calories are given only per 100 g and this can be misleading. For example, when prepared, readymade noodles could have 131 kcal per 100 g but the serving size is 300 g, meaning that it is actually 393 kcal worth of energy. Just to make it more confusing, the weight of the product (before preparation) is only 89 g!

Consider this: low fat milk has more fat than slimline milk. Lean mince has more fat than premium mince.

A word of caution—the nutritional information can be grossly incorrect. One particular noodle product I found claimed to have only 120 kcal per 100 g, where in reality it had 360 kcal per 100 g. If the labelling on a food product is found to be wrong or misleading, the authorities contact the supplier and enforce corrective action. However, as there are usually no fines or legal prosecutions involved, 'misleading through mistake' is just too easy, so be careful.

An interesting section of food labelling is medicinal claims. The labelling cannot make a claim of preventing, treating or curing a human disease. If it does, it is then considered a medicine and falls under different regulations. An exception to this is functional foods that provide additional health benefits.

Examples of these would be cholesterol-lowering margarines and probiotic yoghurts. These claims can be made only if fully justified by medical trials. The actual effect of these types of products is minimal and they may have other undesirable ingredients. For example, a certain margarine may claim to be able to lower your cholesterol by up to 10 per cent, but this is seldom enough by itself to lower your cholesterol to a healthy level. These products can also contain trans-fatty acids, which are best avoided in a healthy diet.

The next major misconception is flavour. If it doesn't clearly say it contains it, it probably doesn't. A label like 'strawberry flavoured' is likely to contain something concocted in a laboratory rather than strawberries. The same goes for cheese, onion, beef, raspberry, lemon, orange or apple flavoured—the list is endless. The key word is 'flavoured' and this is a signal that it's not the real thing. Additives (flavourants, colorants) are usually shown on a label as an 'E Number', but they are not all bad! For example, E101 is Riboflavin, a B vitamin that gives a bright yellow colour.

As for the ingredients list, many ingredients have different names. Some of the more common ones to be aware of would be:

- **FAT—also called vegetable oil, hydrogenated oil, butter, lard, suet, non-dairy fat, cream, sunflower oil, saturated fats and trans fats. All these are fats, all contain calories and they have all been related to some form of illness. They also occur in almost everything we eat and are impossible to avoid. To complicate things, trans fats do not have to be on the label. Your aim should be to be aware of this and reduce all fats in your diet.**

- **SUGAR—can come in the form of sucrose, dextrose, glucose, fructose, maltodextrins, honey, golden syrup, molasses and treacle. Again, even though all these contain energy, some of them are far sweeter than others, which means you need far less of them to get the same effect. For example, fructose (fruit sugar) has a Glycaemic Index of 22 whereas glucose has a Glycaemic Index of 100. Fructose also has a very sweet effect so you will use less of it.**

- **SALT—can be called sodium chloride, MGS NaCl, celery salt or sea salt.**

Let's take a look at a few examples.

We will start with a very obvious comparison between a 'normal' and a 'light' yoghurt.

Normal yoghurt	Light yoghurt
125 g	120 g
136.25 kcal/pot	64 kcal/pot
Protein 5.5 g	Protein 5.2 g
Carbohydrates 21.5 g	Carbohydrates 10.5 g of which sugars 9.6 g
Fat 3.13 g	Fat 0.1 g
	Fibre 0.9 g

As usual, the pot volumes are different; at least in this case it's only by a few grams. The big difference is that the normal yoghurt has more than twice the calories of the light yoghurt. The extra calories would be from the carbohydrates (double the amount, about 46 kcal) and the fat (30 times more, about 27 kcal). The light yoghurt also has a bit of fibre that adds to the daily requirement. No doubt the normal yoghurt will taste creamier and be more satisfying but you pay for this in calories.

A less obvious comparison is that of two typical cereals preferred by children.

Wheat biscuit (crunchy honey)	Cornflakes (sugar coated)
143 kcal/40 g serving	148 kcal/40 g serving
Protein 3.9 g	Protein 1.8 g
Carbohydrates 29.9 g of which sugars 9.8 g	Carbohydrates 34.8 g of which sugars 16 g of which starch 18.8 g
Fat 0.9 g of which saturates 0.2 g	Fat 0.2 g of which saturates 0.04 g
Fibre 3.0 g	Fibre 0.8 g
Sodium 0.2 g	Sodium 0.3 g

Both have similar calories but the carbohydrates are very different. The cornflakes may have 0.7 g less fat but this is put to shame by having over 6 g more sugar. This will increase its Glycaemic Index and, with less fibre, will not give that feeling of fullness.

What concerns me more here is the serving size. Try this for yourself—pour an average bowl of cornflakes or a similar cereal and then weigh it. Surprised? A typical serving size is about 80 g, double the indicated serving size. And in many cases one bowl would not be filling enough. It's quite easy to get through one or two bowls of cornflakes, but it's a lot of chewing getting a bowl of wheat biscuits down. This is where the fibre helps. Typically, more fibre means more chewing, more chewing means a greater feeling of fullness and so eating less.

Approved health claims

- **Low fat/95% fat free**
  For a product to be labelled as low fat, it must contain less than 5 g of fat per 100 g of product.

- **Low in saturated fat**
  Must have less than 3 g of saturated fat per 100 g of product.

- **Virtually fat free**
  Must have minimum 25 per cent less fat than a standard product in its range.

- **Low sugar**
  Less than 5 g per 100 g of product.

- **Sugar free**
  Does not contain any added or naturally occurring sugar.

- **No added sugar**
  No sugar has been added to the product but it contains naturally occurring sugar.

- **Reduced sugar**
  Must have minimum 25 per cent less sugar than a standard product in its range.

- **High fibre**
  Must contain at least 6 g of fibre per 100 g of product.

- **Reduced salt**
  Must have minimum 25 per cent less sodium (salt) than a standard product in its range.

- **Low calorie/diet**
  Must have less than 40 calories in 100 g or 100 ml of product.

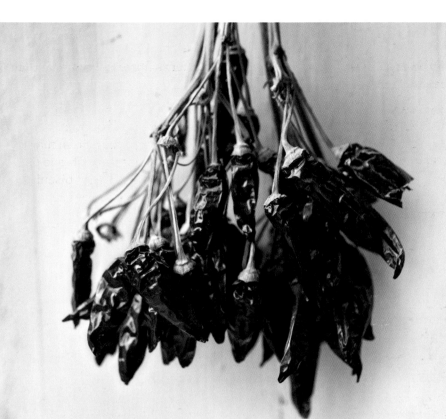

Chapter 4:
Behaviour modification

HABITS, GOOD OR bad, are formed by repetition and eating habits are no exception. Behaviour modification really means changing your behaviour—in this case in relation to eating. As well as cutting out bad habits, it is important to establish new good habits that, with repetition, will eventually become part of your everyday life. The most successful long-term changes in eating habits result from behaviour modification and through this we can create a change in diet and physical activity. It is well known that it is impossible to achieve permanent weight loss without behaviour modification. Behaviour modification takes time and is not an easy process. These known techniques are possible for anybody to implement if they are determined to make a change. They consist of the following.

STIMULUS CONTROL
• Eating three regular meals daily.

• Slowing the pace of eating.

• Shopping for food according to a list and not when hungry.

• Storing food out of sight.

• Separating eating from other activities (e.g. watching TV or reading).

• Eating at the table when at home.

SELF-MONITORING
• Keeping a food and exercise diary.

• Monitoring triggers for overeating and depression.

• Regular monitoring of body weight.

REINFORCEMENT
• Rewarding changes in behaviour, not changes in weight.

SOCIAL SUPPORT
• Selecting a support partner.

• Having a reciprocal agreement (both parties gain from the plan—win-win)

The Diet Diary

We can't expect a change if we carry on doing things in the same way we have done for years. So, if you want that weight to go and stay off, you have to change and to do this you need to know what needs to be changed. Eating is such a common thing that we don't usually pay attention to it or have an exact picture of what we are eating on a daily basis.

I have heard far too many people complain about how little they eat and that they are still putting on weight. It's always about how little I had for breakfast and how light my dinner was. Where does this opinion come from and why do we think that what we eat is very little? How do we create an understanding of what is a normal daily food intake?

My feeling is that portion size and the whole concept of food has become distorted. We are continuously targeted by advertisements and reminded to have a snack and an energy boost. Pub and restaurant portion sizes are huge but because this is what other people eat, we consider this normal. People sometimes compare their quantities with what somebody who is slim is eating without knowing how much this person is eating over the course of a whole week. You see this person eating a lot in that moment, but they might have very little during the rest of the day. You also don't know if this person is already putting on weight and you have just not noticed yet. As I said on p.7, in general, people put on weight.

Another important thing that is forgotten is that we don't consider the energy density of foods. In other words, large quantities of low energy density foods can be eaten without weight gain and will fill you up, whereas only one chocolate muffin, which is very energy rich, meaning it contains a lot of calories, will not fill you.

This is where the diet diary comes in. This is a very helpful and simple exercise with exceptional results.

It's time to open your eyes!

You might now be thinking 'but I can tell you exactly what I eat every day, so what's the point?' You can learn so many things about yourself and the food you eat by keeping this diary—so let's start learning!

TIME TO START YOUR DIET DIARY!

It is important that you record what you eat not only on your working days but also on your days off as people eat and react very differently in different situations. Now start writing down everything you eat for the next week. It is very tempting to say in the morning rush that you will remember and write things down later, but it's too easy to forget and not do it properly, so you are already missing the point of this exercise. You have to write things down immediately and don't cheat! Try to give as much detail about your food quantity and quality as you can. Other things like your environment (are you alone or with a friend or at work) all matter. How hungry were you or was it the visual stimulation of seeing a bar of chocolate on a till counter? If you eat a lot, it might be very difficult to write it all down but don't be ashamed or embarrassed by it.

What usually happens is that people start cutting down immediately and instead of having two biscuits at tea-time they take only one. That's fine, but please write down either with a different colour pen or on one side of the paper what things you have cut down on and how you are changing. Some of the changes you are aware of and some changes happen subconsciously.

Remember the four rules for keeping your diet diary:

- **NOW: Write foods down immediately after they go into your mouth. Any omission will make your record less accurate.**

- **EVERYTHING: Record food and drink—anything that you consume.**

- **CHANGES: Note any changes in eating—your mood and what's around you.**

- **DETAIL: The more detail you give about your food, the more information you will get out of your diary.**

For example:

Time	Consumption	Mood/Environment
10am	Tea with 1 sugar and 2 biscuits	Felt tired before tea
11:30am	340 ml soft drink	
1pm	2 slices white bread with cheese and ham, coffee with 2 sugars, 125 g yoghurt	At work—starving before lunch—tired after, need chocolate
	2 small chocolates	
3pm	Chocolate bar 45 g and coffee with 1 sugar	This gave me a boost

The reason you keep a diet diary is not to criticise yourself, but rather to know what you are doing so that you can learn a different way of doing things. You want to learn how to avoid things and change your behaviour in certain situations. But most of all you want to know what you are doing wrong so you can correct it and start living a healthy life.

The diet diary has six main aims:

1. Increase your food awareness
The first aim of keeping a Diet Diary is to help you discover your level of food forgetfulness. You need to become aware of your food. At the end of the week you will be able to go back and see what changes you made and how much weight you lost with such a small change.

2. Establish a mealtime pattern (eating pattern)
Some people don't have time to have breakfast or don't feel hungry in the morning—the most obvious reason for this is overeating the night before. In their mind they feel that this is a natural and easy way of cutting down on food quantities and calories. They might have something later in the morning, maybe

during morning tea break. At this stage they are usually quite hungry and might eat more, or be less selective about food choice, particularly in the company of work colleagues or friends. They are distracted by conversation and are more likely to eat more than is needed. A mealtime pattern is very important.

3. Record your thoughts and feelings (before and after eating)
Do you get enough sleep and rest? Do you know that tired people eat more and get frustrated more easily? Your feelings and thoughts influence your reactions and ultimately your calorie intake. You need to become aware of your food and the way you react and behave in different situations. You will learn to change your behaviour when you can recognise a pattern that you want to break and substitute a new behaviour or thought.

4. Monitor your hunger and visual stimulation
A lot of things influence our eating. Sensory stimulation is one of the strongest. This was proven almost 100 years ago by Pavlov. Every time he fed a dog, he rang a bell. After a few weeks it was enough to ring the bell to make the dog's salivary glands excrete saliva. In the same way you associate different things with food. While paying for your petrol you see the chocolate bars and you buy one. If you repeat this action many times, eventually just seeing a petrol station makes you feel like having your favourite bar. Unfortunately, modern society is continuously trying to make us eat. Travelling in a bus we see food adverts around us, at home the TV gives us continuous visual reminders of different food options, many of which promise you a lighter figure.

Examine your diet diary: do you always reach for food when you arrive home after a long day's work? While preparing or waiting for dinner are you snacking on something, crisps, toast with some cheese? Did you forget to eat in the afternoon? It's now 6:30 pm, are you starving? Are you used to eating when you relax?

5. Record your daily calorie load
If you write down your food quantities in measurable terms, like grams or millilitres, you should be able to count your total daily calorie consumption. You could see how many of your calories are spent on processed food and how many on natural home-cooked food, how many unhealthy snacks you consume and what you associate with them.

6. Establish how balanced your diet is
Are you getting enough of the right food groups in your diet? For example, do you get enough calcium? What about your fruit and vegetable consumption—do you consume 600 g a day? Does your diet include 25–35 g of fibre a day?

Eat regularly

Timing is everything and this applies to eating as well as other important things in life. Keeping your blood sugar levels stable means avoiding 'starving periods' where blood sugars drop. Maintain stable blood sugars by eating at regular intervals. It is better to eat smaller quantities of the right foods often than a lot in one go. Don't let more than 5 hours pass between your main meals and make sure you have a piece of fruit halfway between them.

Long intervals without eating will make you more vulnerable and your food choices will be governed by extreme hunger (due to low blood sugar levels) and not by rational decisions. We are also more inclined to get easily frustrated when our body is not equipped with enough energy.

A very practical and simple tip is to keep a bag of apples and a bottle of water in your car and an apple in your handbag or briefcase. If you are in a rush and have no time for a healthy lunch, or you are sitting in a traffic jam biting your nails from starvation and frustration, the temptation to stop at a petrol station for a quick chocolate bar is huge, but an apple and some water will get you a long way.

Plan your meals

Planning is important in any project, but it is of vital importance in changing your eating behaviour. Sensible eating requires planning. The food you are supposed to eat—as well as the food you should avoid—first have to be purchased in order to be available for consumption. If you have decided that you are going to reduce or cut crisps from your diet, then these foods should not be kept in the house.

On the other hand, if you are going to increase vegetables in your diet, then you should have them in your house. So behaviour modification starts in the shop with your food choices. One behavioural change reinforces the next one. Before going to the shop you should plan your shopping list and buy only what is on the list. You should also plan to shop after a meal and not just before the next one.

Focus on eating

How much you eat is also influenced by the speed at which you eat your meal and by the attention you give to the moment. The environment is of crucial importance. Eating a bar of chocolate or packet of crisps while driving is wasting calories. Tea and biscuits in the company of work colleagues can become several biscuits before you even notice.

If you realise from your diet diary that snacks and chocolate form a big part of your daily calories and you have always found it very difficult to get rid of this habit, my advice would be the same as that I gave to one woman who was very depressed about her lack of self-control when it came to chocolate.

She could not drive home from work without stopping at the nearby petrol station and buying two bars of chocolate, which she ate on the way home. We decided that the following week the only change she was going to make was that she was not allowed to eat the chocolate in the car but only when she arrived home and sat down to enjoy them. I made sure that she was not trying to make any other changes. The psychological reassurance that she would still get the bars with only a slight delay between the act of buying and the moment of consuming made her succeed.

I know it sounds terribly simple but it's changes like this that will make a big difference to the way we start seeing things. Once you reassure yourself that you can follow through with your first decision, it helps to make the subsequent changes easier. In this patient's case, she told me that once she got home, she felt that one bar was enough and in this way we slowly changed how important chocolate was to her.

Do you eat quickly? Eating quickly is very common and not good for many reasons. Research has indicated that it takes approximately 20 minutes for the message to travel from your stomach to the satiety centre in the brain. This means that if you eat quickly, you might still be eating but in reality you are already full. So take the time to enjoy your food and don't fill your plate again. Are you eating because you are hungry or did you simply like the taste?

Many people have got used to eating in front of the television, which takes the focus off your food. Give full attention to your meal and don't do anything else at the same time. It is so important that we teach this to our children as well. How often do we see children walking or playing while eating?

Exercise

Exercise alone is a very ineffective way of losing weight. I feel its role in weight loss can be overemphasised. Although it is possible to lose weight without exercise, trying to lose weight only by exercising (without dietary change) will give very limited results.

If done in combination with a diet, exercise accounts for approximately 10 per cent of your weight loss success if your BMI falls in the overweight category. For a heavier starting weight (meaning obese Class I to morbidly obese), it can vary from 15 to 20 per cent.

One of the best ways to understand the effect of exercise on calorie usage is by comparing the following:

- **One average chocolate bar contains about 300 kcal.**
- **One hour of low activity such as watching TV burns 70 kcal.**
- **One hour's walk or 30 minutes of aerobic exercise burns around 300 kcal.**

So, without exercise it takes about 4.5 hours to burn up the chocolate bar, or this could also be achieved with 30 minutes of aerobics. It's probably easier to simply not eat the bar in the first place!

In order to lose 1 kg you need to burn 7,500 kcal of energy reserves—equivalent to 25 aerobic sessions. You can see that your food intake is the cornerstone of your weight-loss regime.

BENEFITS OF EXERCISE

I find exercise very beneficial. It helps to ease my frustration, relieve my stress and increase my happy hormones by producing endorphins (hormones of wellbeing). It also helps to keep me toned and burns calories.

First, we should distinguish between day-to-day activity levels and sport exercise.

Sport exercise is a planned, time-specific activity and is generally goal-orientated. In contrast, day-to-day activity is generally unavoidable and specific to your lifestyle.

Although a session of sport can burn a substantial number of calories in a short period of time, changing your lifestyle and general activity levels can have a significantly higher and more sustainable impact. The way we do things is personality related, but we can learn to burn more calories. This is probably best explained through a few examples: I use a lot of 'body language' when communicating with others. I tend to move quickly or run if I forget something in another room or my car. I am impatient and usually do things myself instead of asking and waiting for others to help. Some people always tend to be in a rush and they are definitely using up energy. Do you walk to the shops around the corner or take the car? Do you clean your own house (thoroughly) or do you get help? What about the gardening? You would be surprised how many calories all these activities add up to over the course of a day.

So, if we can increase our energy usage through daily activity change, why bother about exercise? Well, when you do a session of high level activity or sport, your endorphin levels go up and this makes you feel good. It will help motivate you in maintaining your lifestyle changes and you will feel less frustrated. Sport does stimulate appetite, so make sure you drink a lot of water to suppress this and don't reward yourself with a chocolate bar.

The most important reason to exercise is to maintain your lean muscle mass. Unfortunately, when you lose weight, part of this weight loss comes from lean muscular mass. You cannot avoid it, but exercise combined with sufficient protein intake will minimise this muscular loss. Being active, your body needs its muscles and tries to improve them, so naturally the excess calories are then taken out of fat storage.

Being overweight stretches the skin and creates bulges where you don't want them. To flatten these you need to tighten the muscles in that area and also tighten the skin. This can be done only through exercise. In extreme cases, the skin is overstretched and cosmetic surgery would be required to remove the excess.

Exercise will help to reduce high blood pressure and is vitally important for diabetics to reduce their blood sugar levels.

BEGINNING YOUR ACTIVITY ROUTINE

I never push my obese patients to exercise at the beginning of their weight-loss programme because I believe that increased exercise will come naturally once the weight loss is well underway. First get the diet sorted, get used to your new eating habits. Then start including some exercise in your routine, like walking, or using the stairs instead of a lift at work, and slowly build on it until it becomes a normal daily activity like brushing your teeth.

Deciding at which point to start exercising depends to a large degree on your initial starting BMI (refer to Chapter 2). At Class II obesity level any exercise is very strenuous . You feel exhausted and breathless very quickly and it could sometimes even be considered detrimental for your osteoarticular system, specifically your knees and back not to mention your heart. Obviously swimming would be the best type of exercise for anybody regardless of their starting weight. An obese person is actually quite 'fit' as every action requires weight lifting. As they lose the weight, they should find it easier to move simply because there is less weight to move.

Day-to-day activity has decreased nationwide—we use our car to travel even small distances, take the lift instead of the stairs and have numerous appliances and tools to do our work for us. When someone is Class II or morbidly obese, their day-to-day activity levels are even lower. For these individuals, it is unwise to recommend sport exercise at the beginning of their weight-loss plan. I usually advise starting to increase day-to-day activity only when BMI levels fall significantly and the patient starts feeling comfortable with 30 minutes of planned walking a day. This is slowly increased to 90 minutes at least 2–3 times a week. Patients who fall into the overweight or borderline obese levels need to get a minimum 1 hour of brisk walking a day or 1 hour of slow running at least 3 times a week.

The total energy burnt during exercise is quite small but increased exercise will be of vital importance in the weight-loss maintenance phase. The intention should be to create a new active lifestyle that will increase the lean muscle mass and strength and enable the person to burn more energy even at rest. Lean muscle uses energy even at rest so higher lean muscle percentage will increase your resting metabolic rate. In other words you can eat more and maintain your weight. This is vitally important especially for small (short in height) women.

The bottom line is that you are never going to get a flat tummy just by eating the right foods. However, you can lose weight without exercise.

I don't advise patients following a very low calorie diet to do strenuous cardiovascular activity because the carbohydrate intake is low. Muscle uses carbohydrates for instant energy and it does not need insulin for this. This is why insulin-dependent Type 1 and 2 diabetics need to start reducing their insulin injections when their exercise levels go up.

Some common questions I have been asked in relation to exercise include the following.

IS IT TRUE THAT YOUR BODY STARTS BURNING FAT ONLY AFTER 30 MINUTES OF EXERCISE?
No.

When you are on a diet, you are consuming fewer calories than your body needs. The shortfall is made up by using the body's stored reserves, i.e. fat. When doing exercise, more calories are used, but where they come from (food eaten or stored fat) will depend on when and what you last ate, and a number of other factors. It's more important to look at the overall daily average calorie usage than to go into too much detail about individual activities.

IS IT TRUE THAT EXERCISE INCREASES APPETITE?
Yes.

Especially after strenuous exercise you might get sweet cravings because your blood sugar levels are low. Make sure that you drink water after exercise and don't reward yourself with sweet things, rather have some fruit (apple, orange).

IF I EXERCISE A LOT, IS IT TRUE THAT MY WEIGHT MIGHT INCREASE?
Yes.

While your body tones, your lean muscle increases. Lean muscle weighs more than fat tissue so you might feel your clothes getting looser while the scale shows the same number. However, you cannot increase your lean muscle more than a few kilograms a year so you don't have to worry, especially if you are a woman, that you will get too muscular.

Chapter 5:
Step by step to a new lifestyle

BEFORE YOU BEGIN your new lifestyle and weight-loss programme, it is important that you prepare yourself mentally for the changes. Your new lifestyle also requires physical tools and equipment and you need to equip your home accordingly. Don't worry, you don't need to buy everything in one go, but some investment is needed. Otherwise you will find your new routine very time-consuming and you will struggle to follow the instructions.

10 STEPS

1. Face the numbers—what are your BMI and waist measurement? (See Chapter 2 p.7.)

2. Write down why you want to lose weight.

3. Set yourself a realistic goal. I suggest about 10 per cent of weight loss in 12 weeks.

4. Plan your eating and exercise routine for the next 2 weeks. Again, be realistic and write it down.

5. Have a health check-up and get your bloods done (see p.74).

6. Raid your kitchen and give it a health check (more on this later in the chapter).

7. Explore new areas of exercise, e.g. running clubs can be very sociable. Try kick boxing. I recently tried belly dancing, then pole dancing and loved both.

8. Sleep well.

9. Treat yourself and reward your success.

10. Choose a phase that suits your plan (more on this later in the chapter).

DR EVA'S CUPBOARD ESSENTIALS

Before you get going it might be worth investing in some essential sauces and spices that are commonly used in many of my recipes:

1 Balsamic vinegar
2 Chinese five spice
3 Curry powder
4 Fat free vinaigrette
5 Galangal
6 Garlic
7 Kaffir lime leaves
8 Light coconut milk
9 Light spray oil
10 Low fat soft spread cheese, e.g. Philadelphia Light or Laughing Cow
11 High fibre cracker bread, e.g. Finn Crisp or Ryvita
12 Soy sauce
13 Vegetable stock or powder, e.g. Swiss vegetable vegan bouillon
14 Thai red, green, yellow curry paste
15 Thai lemongrass
16 Tom yum paste
17 Turmeric
18 Good quality olive oil
19 Bay leaves
20 Cans of whole peeled tomatoes

HELPFUL HINTS

- If using garlic, store in a cool, dry place but not in the fridge. Did you know that garlic is a natural antibiotic.

- If using curry pastes from a jar, store in the fridge upon opening.

- Fresh lemongrass can be kept, loosely wrapped, in the bottom part of the fridge for up to one week.

- For convenience, coriander can be used in the ground form.

COOKING UTENSILS

- Cast-iron wok: used in most recipes. It is worth investing in a good quality wok as it will retain heat. It will also last for years!

- Garlic crusher: an essential!

- Measuring jugs (100 ml, 500 ml)

- Weighing scales: essential to get your portions correct

- Chopping board—preferably different ones for meat, fish and vegetables

- Good quality sharp knives: can reduce the preparation time

- Kitchen scissors

Learning how to cook healthy food is essential. Prepare one of my filler soups (see the Soups section on p.191) and make sure you always have one pot in the fridge. If you have done this, you have also fulfilled one of the behaviour modification requirements (preparing beforehand to avoid relapses).

Following a healthy diet and lifestyle can help prevent:

- Obesity
- Heart disease
- High cholesterol
- High blood pressure
- Cancer
- Stress
- Poor energy levels
- Constipation
- Infertility
- Depression

A GUIDE TO THE PHASES

This book provides four different diet and recipe plans—all based on specific calorie counts.

Each phase is different and suitable for different lifestyles and weight-loss requirements so which phase should you follow?

Phase 1: 800 kcal—Chapter 6

This is the ketogenic part of the diet. Through a reduction in your carbohydrate intake the body goes into ketosis or 'fat-burning' mode. This phase is most suitable for people who have a BMI >35 (obese Class II) or above, but can also be used for lower BMIs as a short, quick start phase. It could be followed for approximately 10–14 days. It results in quick initial weight loss, which will provide you with the motivation and encouragement you need to continue with your plan. In two weeks a woman can expect to lose approximately 4 kg (9 lb) and a man can expect to lose 6.3 kg (14 lb). Phase 1 should not be followed if you have any serious medical conditions (please see Phase 1 section for full list). No exercise (other than gentle walking) is advised on this plan.

Phase 2: 1,200 kcal—Chapter 8

This phase is suitable as an initial plan for anyone who has a BMI >30 (obese Class I). Alternatively it can be used as a follow-on diet for those who have followed Phase 1. This phase is based on healthy eating guidelines, but carbohydrate and calories have been reduced to incur weight loss. A woman will lose approximately 1–1.5 kg (2.2–3.3 lb) per week depending on size and activity levels. A man can expect to achieve slightly quicker results at 1.5–2.5 kg (3.3–5.5 lb) per week, again depending on size and activity levels. Phase 2 incorporates behaviour modification to help you change your eating patterns to aid long-term weight maintenance once you have reached your goal weight. Exercise should be incorporated into your lifestyle while on this phase.

Phase 3: 1,600 kcal—Chapter 10

This phase is suitable for anyone who has a BMI of 25–29 (overweight) and wishes to achieve a healthy weight. It is suitable as an initial plan for anyone who does regular exercise and can afford to eat more calories and still lose weight. It can also be used as a follow-on diet for anyone who has followed Phase 2. Phase 3 can be used as a maintenance plan for women who are petite (short in height) who would gain weight on a 2,000 kcal diet. Phase 3 is similar to Phase 2 except that portions and calories are increased. Women can expect to lose between 0.6–1 kg (2.2 lb) a week and men can expect to lose up to 1.6 kg (4 lb) a week, in combination with regular exercise.

Phase 4: 2,000 kcal—Chapter 12

This is the maintenance stage and everyone should progress to this to maintain their goal weight. It can be suitable as an initial plan for a man who does strenuous exercise regularly and wants to lose weight gradually at 0.5 kg (1 lb) per week. Note it should not be used as a maintenance plan for petite women (see Phase 3). This phase is based on healthy eating guidelines.

Recipes for all the phases

All phases include delicious recipes for breakfast, lunch and dinner. The recipes include the calorie count so that by choosing one breakfast, one lunch and one dinner from your phase each day you will not have to count calories. However, although meals for each stage of the day are within the same calorie count option, some are slightly higher than others. Make wise choices when choosing your meals, particularly on Phase 1 where carbohydrate count is also important. Calorie and carbohydrate counts are on the Phase 1 recipes so if you do choose a high carbohydrate or calorie at some stage in the day, choose a recipe lower in both for another meal so that you do not exceed your daily allowance.

Snacks

You can also choose snacks daily based on the following:

Phase 1: Choose 2 of the 50 kcal snacks daily

Phase 2: Choose either 3 of the 50 kcal snacks in Phase 1 or 1 of the 150 kcal snacks daily

Phase 3: Choose 2 of the 150 kcal snacks daily

Phase 4: Choose 2 of the 150 kcal snacks daily and 1 of the 50 kcal snacks if needed

I hope you achieve your weight loss goals and enjoy my recipes. If you have any medical concerns or past medical history, it is advisable to see your GP before starting this diet.

Metric conversion charts

Volume measurements		Oven temperatures		
		Fahrenheit	Centigrade	Gas mark
¼ tsp ....1 ml		350° ....180° 4		
½ tsp ....2 ml		375° ....190° 5		
1 tsp...............5 ml		400° ....200° 6		
1 dessertspoon (2 tsp)...............10 ml		425° ....220° 7		
1 tbsp (3 tsp)...............15 ml		450° ....230° 8		

Chapter 6:
Phase 1—ketogenic diet <800 kcal

What is Phase 1?

THE PHASE 1 PLAN is based on consuming less than 800 kilocalories (kcal) a day.

However, it is important to note that this phase of the diet is not based solely on energy deficit (see Chapter 2). We are also aiming to limit carbohydrate foods, which produce the body's easiest form of energy (glucose), to less than 50 g. By doing this, the body is forced to utilise fat stores as energy. Fat is taken to the liver and ketone bodies are produced, a process known as ketosis. This may sound dangerous but it is actually a natural process. This system has been used in Scandinavian countries to treat people in obesity clinics in university hospitals. There is a lot of research to back up the safety of this process.

This phase is effective because ketone bodies act as a very powerful appetite suppressant. This means that the dieter should never feel hungry or deprived and as a result is not tempted to indulge. Ketone bodies also have a psychotonic effect, which means that the dieter should experience a feeling of wellness. An additional benefit is that the dieter usually feels their energy levels increasing because the body has found another source of energy.

The meal options in Phase 1 are based primarily on vegetables, mainly those that grow above the ground, and are very low in carbohydrates (cabbage, courgettes, cauliflower, mushrooms, broccoli, celery, etc.—see the list). Vegetables that are not allowed, such as onion, garlic (only a small amount used for flavour in my recipes) and carrots, are too high in carbohydrate and should be avoided to induce ketosis. The recipes feature lean protein sources such as eggs, chicken, turkey, fish and red meat. As already stated, carbohydrate intake needs to be kept to less than 50 g a day. This is actually harder to achieve than it may seem. Apart from the allowed vegetables, all other carbohydrate foods need to be eliminated from the diet. Obvious sources of high carbohydrates to avoid include fruit, cereals, bread, rice, pasta, confectionery, juice, fizzy and sugary drinks. Less obvious sources of carbohydrate that should also be avoided are milk and dairy products, sauces, certain vegetables, mints and chewing gum. Be aware of products that state the contents are sugar free, e.g. many chewing gums—they still actually contain carbohydrates.

The adequate protein intake will provide the body with a sufficient supply of protein for its essential needs. As a result, the body's lean muscle mass is protected, preventing muscle wastage. The large allowance of a variety of vegetables means you will achieve the recommended daily intake of fibre (25–35 g/day) from a natural source. Vegetables are also a key provider of essential vitamins and minerals to maintain a good nutritional status. However, as this diet excludes some food groups, I recommend also taking a multivitamin that contains calcium to ensure that all of your nutritional needs are being met. Also remember that alcohol is strictly forbidden on this phase because it interferes with the process of ketosis.

Medications

We are continuously offered different types of commercial magic pills to lose weight without any effort. None of them do anything significant. You would waste time and money buying them. The only thing that would get lighter is your wallet! But there is some help available out there. I want to emphasise the word 'help' as this means that you must still make changes and put the effort in.

A pharmacological approach is an accepted form of treatment when a diet and exercise regime on its own has failed. Even though the medication available can provide additional help (and motivation), it is better to change to a new lifestyle naturally and do so without the help of any drugs.

At present there are licensed prescription drugs available for the treatment of obesity with two totally different mechanisms of action.

Some work by stopping a percentage of the dietary fat being absorbed by the body. Its main place of action is the gut, where it prevents about 30 per cent of dietary fat being absorbed. It does not 'melt' the body fat, as many people want to believe. Many patients have found these drugs beneficial because they encourage them to avoid fatty foods and be more vigilant about foods' fat content—the main side effect being an upset tummy if you are not careful.

Other drugs work on the brain, where they attempt to control a patient's eating behaviour. They block some receptors in the brain that would, under normal circumstances, draw the neurotransmitter serotonin back into the cells. When these receptors are blocked, the serotonin/noradrenalin stays out longer. This means that your serotonin or happy hormone levels are higher. The bottom line is that a patient feels fuller quicker, becomes satisfied with smaller portions and is less frustrated or tense.

These drugs have been withdrawn here and in continental Europe due to the side effects being considered dangerous.

Phase 1 is not a long-term solution to weight loss but is purely a kick-start to your diet. Unlike other diets, the suppressed appetite and quick initial weight loss you get with this plan will provide huge motivation and encouragement to continue. I recommend that this phase is followed for 10–14 days in order to get a good psychological boost to make you realise you can lose weight.

Phase 1 should be followed by those wishing to get a quick, initial weight loss to motivate them. This plan is ideal for anybody whose BMI is greater than 35 (obese Class II). The reason for this is that Phase 1 is effective on its own and does not require exercise to aid weight loss. This makes it ideal for anybody who has difficulty exercising due to physical immobility (arthritis, osteoarticular aches and pains) or cardiovascular conditions that would put unnecessary stress on the body, increasing the risk of heart attack or stroke. From a psychological point of view, a lot of people who are obese experience difficulty motivating themselves to diet since they feel they have so much weight to lose. The quick initial weight loss on Phase 1 provides a huge mental boost and encourages continued effort to lose weight.

CAUTION

Phase 1 should not be followed by anyone who does not have proper functioning kidneys because kidneys are essential to deal with the breakdown of fat and protein as well as the excretion of waste from the body. This phase is not recommended for anybody with dia- betes. Please consult your doctor before commencing the plan. I use Phase 1 for people with Type 2 diabetes in my clinics but this is strictly under medical supervision.

Benefits

Apart from the benefits already mentioned, such as the appetite suppressant effect, improved energy levels and a feeling of wellness, this plan introduces a regular eating pattern. It also exercises portion control and introduces vegetables into the diet. The plan highlights the importance of reaching your recommended intake of fibre, which is not usually achieved in an average diet. In two weeks women can expect to lose 4 kg (9 lb) and men can expect to lose 6.3 kg (14 lb).

Side effects

Side effects are usually noticed in the first three days of beginning the diet as the body adapts to using a new energy source. Until this process is complete, you may experience some hunger, dizziness, headaches, tiredness and low energy levels. The side effects usually pass after the first three days, by which time you should be experiencing improved energy levels, a feeling of wellness and diminishing hunger as you enter a state of ketosis. You may experience bad breath (halitosis). This is a sign that your body is burning fat as a main source of energy and the diet is working effectively. You can chew parsley, mint or take special mints to alleviate this.

Exercise

Strenuous exercise should be avoided in Phase 1 because it may leave you feeling weak. However, gentle daily activities may still be carried out.

Eating out

Eating out is still possible on Phase 1. The best options when eating out are lean meat or fish served with vegetables or salad. Fish is the best option because, unlike other meats, restaurants rarely exceed the portion of fish because it is expensive. Therefore you should be able to eat the portion that you get. When choosing vegetables, try to select the lowest in carbohydrate. When choosing salad, avoid creamy salad dressings. Vinegar or oil dressings are the best options. Always ask for dressing on the side. Send the bread basket back to keep temptation at bay. Unfortunately, rice, pasta and potatoes are not permitted—no matter how good they look. As you would expect, alcohol and dessert are not allowed!

General advice for eating out

You can go out and enjoy the evening without destroying your weight-loss progress. Simply learn to choose carefully and avoid certain things.

The basic rules of eating out:

- Never go out starving.
- Eat light but filling food during the day.
- Eat something before you go, like a low calorie homemade vegetable soup, or have an apple on your way (depending on the phase you are following) and drink water.
- Avoid pre-dinner snacks like peanuts, crisps and bread from the basket.
- If there are vegetable snacks like carrot and celery sticks, nibble on these.
- Exercise moderation with alcohol—no diet can work if you drink too much. Avoid it or at least alternate every second drink with water on a unit basis (1 unit of alcohol relates to 1 glass of water).
- Stick to protein- and fibre-rich vegetables and very few carbohydrates (potatoes, rice, pasta).
- Avoid deep fried and especially batter-covered foods.
- Eat slowly—try to be the last to finish.
- Don't feel obliged to eat everything on your plate.
- You don't have to miss out on courses, just choose sensibly.

People don't tend to notice what you are eating but they do notice if you're not 'joining in' and this could result in an uncomfortable situation.

Which cuisine to choose?

ITALIAN
Very easy to eat light! Instead of choosing a pasta or rice dish, choose a *Minestrone di verdura*, which is a type of vegetable soup. Italians love their green salads and they should always be on the menu. Ask for the salad dressing on the side and use it with extreme moderation.

Antipasto misto is a good starter. It includes a variety of cold meats but don't touch the salamis.

Grilled fish is always a safe and tasty option and all tomato-based sauces are lower in calories. Usually chicken dishes are cooked in tomato, e.g. *Pollo alla cacciatore*. Veal is a real Italian favourite. Tasty *Saltimbocca alla romana* is a good source of protein but remember to order it with steamed vegetables and not garlic or creamy potatoes.

INDIAN
Many starters are deep fried or covered in batter and fried so avoid these. A chicken skewer or grilled prawns are fine but go easy on the sauces. Alternatively, you could ask for a salad.

Spicy food is generally filling but avoid diluting the 'burn' with large amounts of rice and bread. Try to choose a 'dry' dish but if it comes with a creamy sauce, don't indulge in the sauce.

There is usually a selection of speciality dishes that includes oven-baked fish or grilled steak.

THAI AND CHINESE

As with Indian, many starters are deep fried so avoid these. Some of the soups can be very light, e.g. *tom yum goong*, and are a good choice. Steamed mussels or salads are also usually on the menu.

For the main course, there is a variety of stir-fried food but try to choose vegetable-based meals and not rice-based ones. Thai cuisine usually has the biggest selection of healthy foods with a good choice of baked meats, salads, vegetables, etc.

MEXICAN

There is a large selection beyond tortillas, enchiladas and tacos. There is a great variety of soups (courgette, tomato, avocado) and interesting vegetables.

Main courses could include peppers stuffed with beans or mince, chilli vegetable dishes, green bean and sweet pepper salad, or a choice of fish and chicken dishes.

Counting calories

Please be aware that 800 calories builds up very quickly and it is very difficult to stay within this limit. Bear in mind that you will be very limited in the foods you eat for this reason. For instance, an average banana has 25 g carbohydrates and 100 kcal. One slice of white toast has an average of 97 kcal and 19 g carbohydrates.

Although the calories of each breakfast, lunch or dinner are similar, small variations do add up and portion size will vary depending on which food you choose due to higher calorie content of some ingredients. It is worth making a little bit of effort in your food preparation to get more from your calories as sometimes the 'easy option' does not get you as far. I have also included the calorie and carbohydrate counts of each meal in Phase 1. If you do choose a higher calorie or higher carbohydrate option at breakfast, lunch or dinner, please choose a lower option at another stage during the day so that overall you will not exceed your 800 calories or 50 g carbohydrates.

Protein should be included in all three meals and snacks. It is hard to define how much in total each serving should provide but you should aim for 0.8 g protein/kg/body weight a day. By including protein-rich sources in meals, you should achieve this.

You should aim to consume your recommended 5 a day or 600 g of vegetables a day (as fruit is not allowed on this plan except for grapefruit and rhubarb) and they should form the basis of your diet.

I have analysed the calorie content of the recipes as exactly as possible using WISP V3.0 (Tinuviel software) but please be aware that figures are approximate.

Meal options

Breakfast 200 kcal, Lunch 200 kcal, Dinner 300 kcal, Snacks less than 50 kcal

Breakfast
1 Thai-style prawn grapefruit cocktail
2 Low carbohydrate Irish breakfast
3 Omelette with feta cheese and vegetables
4 Creamy peppadew mushrooms

Lunch
1 Aubergine crab rolls
2 Broccoli soup with chicken
3 Green curry turnip soup with lemon zest prawns
4 Filled cabbage leaves
5 Warm beef salad, Thai style

Dinner
1 Italian *Bagna Cauda* with grilled green peppers
2 Salmon with roasted vegetables
3 Low carbohydrate tomato aubergine bake
4 Beef and lemongrass stir-fry
5 Chicken stir-fry with ginger and coconut milk
6 Sea bass with stir-fried vegetables
7 Galangal red curry with fish sauce
8 Aubergines stuffed with meat ratatouille

Snacks
Snacks: You can choose 1 mid-morning and 1 mid-afternoon
1 Rhubarb and jelly (see recipe on p.68) (10 kcal)
2 Lemon surprise (see recipe on p.69) (22 kcal)
3 1 packet cheese strings (60 kcal)
4 ½ grapefruit (24 kcal, 5.4 g carbohydrate)
5 2–4 celery sticks with 30 g low fat soft cheese spread (30 g serving is 47 kcal, 1.2 g carbohydrates)
6 Babybel light (42 kcal)
7 2 crab seafood sticks (50 kcal)

Clockwise from top right: warm beef salad, Thai style; galangal red curry with fish sauce; aubergine crab rolls; broccoli soup with chicken; Thai-style prawn grapefruit cocktail; chicken stir-fry with ginger and coconut milk

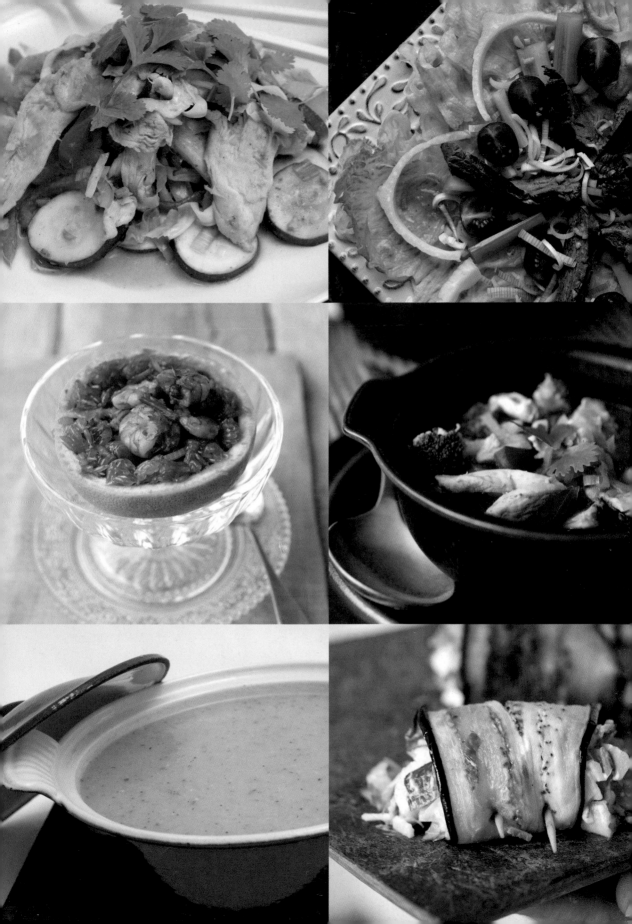

Breakfast recipes

Thai-style prawn grapefruit cocktail

This recipe is a combination of my love for Thai food and inspiration from a starter I ate on one of my trips. Grapefruit is lower in carbohydrates than other fruit and has a high fibre content, which makes it quite filling.

SERVES **2**

1 fresh lemongrass stalk
20 g/3 spring onions
600 g/2 grapefruits
1 tbsp fresh coriander, depending on taste
250 g frozen prawns
$\frac{1}{5}$ tsp hot chilli paste (or fresh chilli, chopped)
10–15 g/4 crushed garlic cloves
2 tbsp soy sauce

HOW TO PREPARE:

1 Cut the end off the fresh lemongrass. Peel off outer layer of damaged leaves if necessary. Cut in 2 cm long strips obliquely, thick enough so that they remain visible and can be removed before eating.

2 Chop spring onion finely.

3 Slice both of the grapefruits through the centre to create 4 halves.

4 Scoop out the contents of the grapefruit using a knife by putting the knife between the outer layer of the flesh and the skin and cut in a circular motion.

5 Chop grapefruit contents finely and empty the contents into a bowl.

6 Chop coriander very finely using a kitchen scissors or a knife and add to bowl.

7 Put a non-stick pan on a medium heat and add frozen prawns.

8 Add lemongrass and spring onions to pan.

9 Mix chilli, crushed garlic and 2 tablespoons of soy sauce and add to pan.

10 Cook until prawns defrosted and chilli and soy sauce have blended together.

11 When the prawns are hot, empty the mixture into the bowl containing the grapefruit and mix together.

12 Scoop mixture into emptied grapefruit halves and serve 2 halves per person.

If you don't want to serve both halves now, you could wrap the 2 halves in cling film, store in the fridge and eat the next day. Each grapefruit half contains 85 calories.

APPROXIMATELY **170** KCAL, 15.4 G CARBOHYDRATE FOR 2 GRAPE-FRUIT HALVES

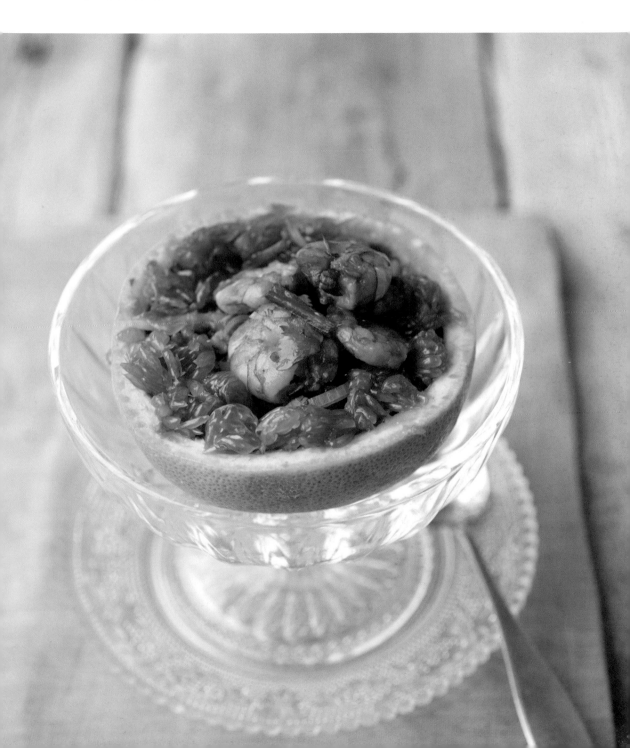

Low carbohydrate Irish breakfast

Everybody in Ireland is addicted to their fries. I know this is not the same as a classic Irish fry up, but it is not bad for the number of calories it contains.

SERVES **1**

200 g turnip
1 egg white
1 tomato, halved and grilled
2 turkey rashers

HOW TO PREPARE:

1   Peel and chop turnip in small cubes.
2   Boil turnip until soft (approximately 20 minutes). When cooked, drain water and mash turnip.
3   Add egg white to pot.
4   Mash together.
5   Line a baking tray with greaseproof paper.
6   Take a scoop of turnip/egg mixture using a spoon and flatten into the shape of a hash brown. You should get 4 hash browns.
7   Place hash browns and tomato halves on the lined baking tray and put on the top shelf of oven at 200 °C.
8   After 7 minutes add the turkey rashers.
9   Leave to cook for approximately 8 minutes (total cooking time approximately 15 minutes depending on the oven). Make sure the rashers are well cooked.
10 Serve rashers, hash browns and tomato together.

APPROXIMATELY **1 3 2** KCAL, 13 G CARBOHYDRATE PER SERVING

Omelette with feta cheese and vegetables

I love feta cheese and this is quick and easy to do. As feta cheese already has salt in it, you do not need to add any. This is extremely filling and, together with vegetables, can be used as a breakfast, lunch or main course. A very versatile meal.

SERVES ❶

150 g broccoli, cut into small florets
2 egg whites
1 egg yolk
2 tbsp water
light spray oil
30 g light feta cheese (contains 30 per cent less fat)
pinch of salt and black pepper

HOW TO PREPARE:

1 Start by steaming your broccoli or alternatively boil it.

2 Whisk egg whites with egg yolk and add water.

3 Lightly oil a non-stick frying pan. Heat pan to medium heat and pour in egg mixture. Cook until the egg becomes firm.

4 Crumble feta cheese with a fork and sprinkle it in the middle of your omelette. Add a pinch of salt and pepper.

5 Once omelette is cooked, turn one half over to melt the cheese.

6 Serve with steamed broccoli.

APPROXIMATELY ❷❶❶ KCAL, 9 G CARBOHYDRATE PER SERVING

Creamy peppadew mushrooms

This is a variation on the classic filled mushrooms with feta cheese and pesto.

SERVES ❶

100 g/3 Portobello mushrooms
30 g/1 slice of ham
30 g ricotta cheese
2 peppadews
1 tbsp soy sauce

HOW TO PREPARE:

1 Pre-heat oven to 200 ˚C.
2 Wash mushrooms and place on a baking tray lined with a large sheet of tinfoil that will be big enough to cover the mushrooms later.
3 Chop a slice of ham finely and mix in a bowl with ricotta cheese.
4 Finely slice 2 peppadews and add them to ham and cheese mixture.
5 Add in a tablespoon of soy sauce and mix well.
6 Using a spoon, fill the mushrooms evenly with the mixture. Close the tinfoil over the mushrooms creating a parcel, but leave some space to allow steam to circulate.
7 Place in the oven for 15 minutes and then serve.

NOTE: You could make this recipe in bulk and eat it cold. This is also a great starter for a low calorie cocktail party!

APPROXIMATELY ❶❶❼ KCAL, 3 G CARBOHYDRATE PER SERVING

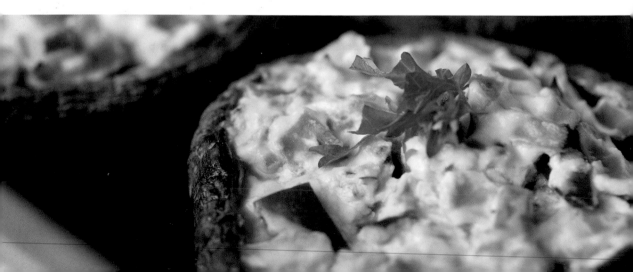

Lunch recipes

Aubergine crab rolls

This is Japanese-style and would be perfect for a cocktail party. It's very high in protein and low in carbohydrate. It also fills you up. It is better to make it the night before in bulk as it is quite laborious.

SERVES ❷

6 ROLLS PER PERSON
400 g/2 good size aubergines
pinch of salt
16 crab sticks
100 ml half fat crème fraîche

1 tsp ready prepared Wasabi
3–4 leaves of butterbean or iceberg lettuce
soy sauce

cocktail sticks

HOW TO PREPARE:

1   Wash 2 aubergines. Chop off both ends. Cut into thin slices lengthways using a slicer.

2   Lay out on a clean surface and sprinkle both sides with salt to draw out the bitter juices.

3   Leave for approximately 20 minutes and then rinse off the salt.

4   Preheat oven to 200 ˚C.

5   Line a baking tray with greaseproof paper.

6   Place aubergine slices on baking tray and bake for 5 minutes. If you overcook the aubergines, you will not be able to roll them.

7   In the meantime, mince crab meat very thinly with a knife.

8   Mix with half fat crème fraîche and Wasabi.

9   Place crab meat mixture evenly on the aubergine slices. This is why it is important to get good size aubergines so that the mixture fits on the slice.

10   Thinly slice lettuce and place on top of the fish mixture and roll the aubergine to enclose all contents. Hold roll in place using a cocktail stick.

11   Put back in the oven for 2–3 minutes to cook them further.

12   Drizzle with soy sauce and serve.

APPROXIMATELY ❷❶❶ KCAL, 16 G CARBOHYDRATE IN 6 ROLLS

Broccoli soup with chicken

I made this soup for a fussy patient with cauliflower to camouflage the taste of broccoli. It went down very well and he learned to eat more vegetables and lost the extra weight.

SERVES ❹–❻

400 g broccoli, chopped in florets
350 g cauliflower, chopped in florets
200 g/4 celery sticks, sliced
150 g/1 leek, sliced thinly
100 g/1 courgette, sliced
2 tbsp soy sauce

1 vegetable stock cube
1 litre boiling water from kettle
1 or 2 garlic cloves
pinch of black or white pepper
240 g cooked chicken pieces

HOW TO PREPARE:

1 Place all vegetables in a large saucepan. Add soy sauce and stock cube dissolved in 1 litre of boiling water from kettle.

2 Add garlic and a pinch of white or black pepper or according to taste.

3 Bring to the boil. Then simmer approximately 20 minutes until vegetables are soft.

4 Add cooked chicken and serve.

5 Liquidise if preferred.

APPROXIMATELY ❶❼❾ KCAL, 8.3 G CARBOHYDRATE PER SERVING

Green curry turnip soup with lemon zest prawns

This is one of my favourite soup recipes that I give out at my clinics. There are a lot of ingredients but it is well worth making. It is a healthy soup and especially good for curry lovers. You can substitute your preferred spice for the curry paste and chilli.

SERVES 8-10

600 g/1 turnip
350 g/3 courgettes
250 g/2 leeks
200 g/½ head of celery
1 tbsp olive oil
1 red chilli, deseeded and chopped
3 garlic cloves, crushed
1 tsp Chinese five spice
1 tbsp Thai green curry paste
2 tbsp fish sauce
1 vegetable stock cube
1–1½ litre boiling water from kettle (depending on how thick you would like the soup)
100 ml light coconut milk
100 g prawns (per person)
1 lemon, squeezed

HOW TO PREPARE:

1 Wash the vegetables. Slice the courgettes, leeks and celery. Chop the turnips into cubes.

2 Heat oil in wok or large pot. Fry chopped turnip, courgettes, leeks and celery for a few minutes. Add chilli, garlic, Chinese five spice, curry paste and fish sauce.

3 Dissolve stock cube with the boiling water from kettle. Add to pot.

4 Simmer for 30–40 minutes or until vegetables are soft.

5 Allow to cool slightly before adding light coconut milk to pot and stir thoroughly.

6 Serve a bowl of soup with 100 g prawns drizzled with lemon juice.

APPROXIMATELY 176 KCAL, 11.5 G CARBOHYDRATE PER SERVING

Filled cabbage leaves

This Russian recipe is very common in Finland, mixed with rice. I've made it with ratatouille to aid weight loss. Cabbage has very few calories but is high in fibre and very filling. You could add red curry paste as the cabbage leaves absorb all the flavour from the ratatouille.

SERVES **4**

YOU WILL GET 24 FILLED CABBAGE LEAVES; 4–5 ROLLS PER PORTION

24 big cabbage leaves (white and green)
100 g/1 large leek
3 celery sticks
1 tbsp olive oil
300 g premium lean minced beef
2 tbsp soy sauce

½ tsp white pepper
2 tsp turmeric
3 garlic cloves, crushed
800 g/2 (400 g) cans of chopped tomatoes
1–2 tsp curry paste (optional, hot)

cocktail sticks

HOW TO PREPARE:

1 White cabbage: Place whole cabbage in a steamer or double boiler for few minutes. This will soften outer leaves and enable you to remove them. After removing 1–2 outer leaves, you need to replace the cabbage in the steamer and repeat this procedure until you have 'peeled' the whole cabbage. Steam 3–4 peeled cabbage leaves at a time until soft enough to use as wraps. This part of the method is the most time-consuming. Be careful not to burn your fingers.

2 Green cabbage: Cut the hard stem off and peel leaves. Stop when leaves are small near the centre, which will be too small to use as wraps. You may need a few cabbage heads this way, but you can shed the remaining small leaves and use them for a soup or a stir-fry! It is a bit quicker to use green cabbage as you can prepare your mince and vegetables while the leaves are steaming.

3 Scrape down stem (hardest part) of leaves until it is flattened. This will make it easier to roll them and close them down with a cocktail stick once filled.

4 Chop the leeks and celery thinly. Heat oil in wok or a big non-stick pan. Add the meat, spices and garlic. Fry until brown. Add vegetables and can of tomatoes. Cook without lid until vegetables are almost soft and excess water has evaporated so that you have obtained a thick sauce. If vegetables and meat are not cooked and start sticking to wok, you can add a little water.

5 While the ratatouille is cooking, prepare cabbage leaves if not done already. It can be useful to steam leaves first so you can let them cool down for easy handling.

6 Divide this ratatouille now between cabbage leaves—don't be greedy, it only takes

a small tablespoon to fill one! Roll them in parcels using cocktail sticks to keep them together. To re-heat, simply place on steamer or microwave if preferred. These are also nice cold.

APPROXIMATELY ❶❽⓿ KCAL, 10 G CARBOHYDRATE PER SERVING

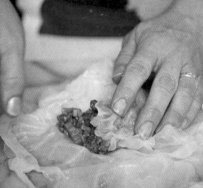

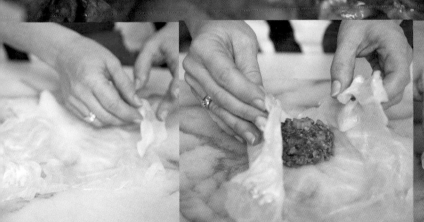

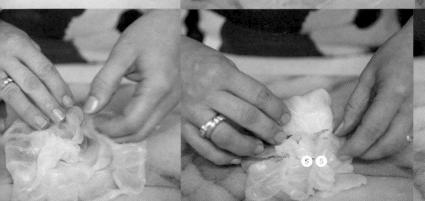

Warm beef salad, Thai style

A patient of mine gave me the idea for this recipe. It is also a good starter option if you are having friends over. It's very tasty and the dressing has a very appealing aroma.

SERVES ④

450 g/1 head broccoli
300 g/1 big fennel
150 g/2 celery sticks
250 g cherry or perrino tomatoes
150 g/1 leek
2 fillet steaks of 120 g each
500 g iceberg lettuce
light spray oil

Salad dressing
3 garlic cloves, crushed
2 cm ginger, peeled and grated
2 tbsp fish sauce
2 tsp low calorie sweetener
¼ tsp Thai red curry paste
juice of 1 lime
2 tbsp orange juice

4 serving dishes

HOW TO PREPARE:

1 Wash the vegetables. Chop the broccoli into florets and cut the fennel, leeks and celery into thin slices.

2 Steam the broccoli for 5 minutes and remove it from the pot when still crunchy.

3 Cook the fillet steaks to your preference in a non-stick frying pan using a small amount of oil (use light spray oil).

4 Divide the lettuce and the rest of the ingredients between the four individual serving dishes. Cut the tomatoes in halves and distribute between the four dishes. Cut the fillet steaks into thin strips and place on top of other ingredients.

5 Prepare the salad dressing by mixing the ingredients in a bowl.

6 Let everybody sprinkle their own salad dressing as it is strong but full of flavour!

APPROXIMATELY ①⑥⑤ KCAL, 8.5 G CARBOHYDRATE PER SERVING

Dinner recipes

Italian *Bagna Cauda* with grilled green peppers

This is a typical recipe from the Piemonte region in Italy, which has a lot of French influence. In fact, you often find the bagna cauda *sauce in southern France with a crudité platter and a boiled egg. This is one of my favourite recipes but watch out — you will smell of garlic the next day!*

SERVES ❷

600 g/4 green peppers
50 g anchovies
2 tbsp olive oil
4–5 garlic cloves
2 tbsp light sour cream
2 eggs

HOW TO PREPARE:

1   Preheat oven to 200 ˚C.

2   Wash peppers and remove core. Cut in half and place peppers outside up in a non-stick oven dish. Place in the top part of the oven for 30 minutes until they become shrivelled and slightly brown.

3   When cooked, place peppers in a glass dish and cover with cling film to keep in the steam. This will make it easier to remove the skin of the peppers. Keep peppers covered until they are cool (approximately 30 minutes).

4   Drain anchovies and place in a small saucepan with olive oil.

5   Peel and crush garlic and add to saucepan.

6   Cook the mixture over a low heat, stirring continuously until it melts into a mush.

7   Remove from the heat and add in the sour cream and whisk until it is creamy.

8   In the meantime, boil 2 eggs.

9   Peel the skin off the peppers using a sharp knife.

10   Place peppers on a plate and cover with sauce.

11   When eggs are boiled, allow to cool and peel off the shell.

12   Crumble the eggs with a fork and spread over the peppers and sauce.

APPROXIMATELY ❸❸❶ KCAL, 3.9 G CARBOHYDRATE PER SERVING

Salmon with roasted vegetables

This is my take on a classic salmon dish. It's quick and easy to make and very tasty.

SERVES **1**

75 g/½ large green pepper
150–200 g/1–2 courgettes
50 g/½ small leek
120 g salmon fillet
light spray oil

sprinkle of lemon pepper
1 tsp chilli flakes
½ lime
coriander to taste

HOW TO PREPARE:

1 Preheat the oven to 200 °C.

2 Wash the vegetables. Cut the pepper and courgette into strips. Slice the leek finely. Place on one side of an oiled oven tray.

3 Place salmon on a large piece of tinfoil. Sprinkle with lemon pepper, chilli flakes and squeeze lime over it. Close tinfoil to create a parcel, leaving enough room on the inside for steam to circulate, and place on the other side of the baking tray.

4 Spray oil over vegetables.

5 Place in oven for 15–20 minutes.

6 Sprinkle coriander over the cooked salmon and serve with vegetables.

APPROXIMATELY **270** KCAL, 8.1 G CARBOHYDRATE PER SERVING

Low carbohydrate tomato aubergine bake

In the original Italian recipe, parmigiana di melanzane, *the aubergines are fried in oil, but cooking them my way greatly reduces the calories without compromising the taste. You can make it for the whole family or freeze it in portions.*

SERVES **4**-**6**

1,100 g/4–5 aubergines
pinch of salt
250 g/1–2 leeks
light spray oil
1 tbsp olive oil
800 g/2 (400 g) cans of whole peeled tomatoes
1 tbsp Swiss vegetable vegan bouillon
black pepper to taste
125 g/1 light mozzarella cheese, grated

HOW TO PREPARE:

1 Preheat oven to 200 ˚C.

2 Slice aubergines about 1 cm thick and salt both sides. Leave aubergines to rest for 15–20 minutes to draw out sour water. Then rinse and place on a baking tray covered with greaseproof paper. Bake in oven for 10 minutes.

3 Wash and slice the leeks.

4 Heat oil in a large non-stick pan and add the leeks. Fry gently for 1–2 minutes.

5 Add the tins of tomatoes, Swiss vegetable vegan bouillon and pepper.

6 Break tomatoes with spoon while cooking.

7 Simmer for 20–40 minutes without a lid so that the water evaporates and a sauce is formed, stirring occasionally.

8 Slightly oil an ovenproof dish using light spray oil. In this dish place a layer of aubergines and then a layer of the tomato sauce. Repeat this layering and finish with a layer of tomato sauce.

9 Cover dish with tinfoil and place in the oven at 200 ˚C for 20–40 minutes.

10 Five minutes before dish is removed from oven, sprinkle with the mozzarella cheese.

APPROXIMATELY **135** KCAL, 9.5 G CARBOHYDRATE PER SERVING

Beef and lemongrass stir-fry

Lemongrass is an ingredient that many people would never use. It is worth getting it fresh as it has a stronger fragrance. When I was living in South Africa I grew it in my garden but I don't think it would survive in Ireland.

SERVES ❶

150 g white cabbage
150 g/1 courgette
100 g/1 small leek
120 g striploin steak
1 tbsp olive oil or light spray oil
¼ tsp tom yum paste or other red curry paste
½ beef stock cube dissolved in 100 ml boiling water
1 tbsp soy sauce
1 lemongrass stalk

HOW TO PREPARE:

1 Chop the cabbage and courgette into thin strips and slice the leek thinly.

2 Cut meat into thin strips, using a pair of sharp scissors or a knife.

3 Spray oil in a wok or a large non-stick pan. Start by first gently browning your beef with the curry paste.

4 Add cabbage, cover and fry for 3 minutes. Then add courgette and leek.

5 Add in stock and soy sauce.

6 Remove the outer layer of lemongrass if required. Slice in two, keeping it in visible strips as it will later need to be removed, add to wok and stir.

7 If ingredients start sticking to the wok, add a little boiling water from kettle.

8 Cook until vegetables are still slightly crunchy.

9 Remove lemongrass before serving.

APPROXIMATELY ❷❾❽ KCAL, 17 G CARBOHYDRATE PER SERVING

Chicken stir-fry with ginger and coconut milk

This is one of the most popular recipes in my clinic and probably has about one-quarter of the calories of a take-away option. It is slightly higher in calories and carbohydrates than some of the other dishes so match it with a low carb and low calorie breakfast and lunch.

SERVES ❶

50 g/½ leek
1 celery stick
100 g/1 courgette
100 g cabbage
75 g/½ large green pepper
150 g chicken breast
light spray oil
1½ cm ginger, grated

2 garlic cloves, crushed
¹/₈ tsp Thai red curry paste
1 tbsp soy sauce
¼ vegetable stock cube
100 ml boiling water from kettle
100 ml light coconut milk
¼ tsp turmeric
fresh coriander to garnish

HOW TO PREPARE:

1   Wash vegetables and cut leek and celery in small half circles. Cut courgette, cabbage and pepper in strips.

2   Cut chicken in small strips.

3   Light spray oil a wok or use a non-stick pan and heat to gently brown the chicken.

4   Then add ginger, garlic, curry paste and soy sauce. Add in all the vegetables, and stir frequently.

5   Melt vegetable stock cube in 100 ml boiling water.

6   Pour in vegetable stock when ingredients start sticking to the wok and reduce heat. Cover and leave to simmer until vegetables and chicken are cooked.

7   Add coconut milk and turmeric. Cover and simmer for further 2–3 minutes, stirring occasionally.

8   Serve with fresh coriander sprinkled over the top.

APPROXIMATELY ❸❸❸ KCAL, 22.5 G CARBOHYDRATE PER SERVING

Sea bass with stir-fried vegetables

This is an excellent recipe to help incorporate fish into your diet. You can have a larger portion of white fish than chicken or meat as it is lower in calories. It's a good option for you if you want more protein on your plate. Too quick and easy to be this tasty!

SERVES **1**

light spray oil
75 g turnip, cut in thin strips
25 g white cabbage, cut into strips
100 g broccoli, cut into small florets
50 g scallions, sliced thinly
1 garlic clove, crushed
boiling water from kettle (approximately 50–100 ml)
1 sea bass fillet (approximately 200 g)
½ lemon
lemon pepper/lemon and pepper seasoning
1 tbsp soy sauce
200 g/½ (400 g) can of whole peeled tomatoes

HOW TO PREPARE:

1 Spray oil in a wok to be used for cooking the vegetables. Allow to heat before adding turnip, white cabbage, broccoli, scallions, and finally garlic to your wok.

2 Pour in boiling water from kettle if vegetables start sticking to the wok. Cover and leave for 1–2 minutes to allow steam to build up. Then remove lid and stir continuously. Repeat this process until vegetables are cooked but still crunchy.

3 Spray oil in a non-stick pan and place on a medium heat. Place sea bass in pan, skin side down. Squeeze the juice of half a lemon over the sea bass and season with lemon pepper seasoning and soy sauce.

4 After 2 minutes turn over sea bass and leave to cook for a further minute. After 1 minute add tin of tomatoes and a splash of water. Turn off hob and leave to steam for a further minute.

5 Dish up vegetables and serve with the sea bass and tomatoes.

APPROXIMATELY **313** KCAL, 16.3 G CARBOHYDRATE PER SERVING

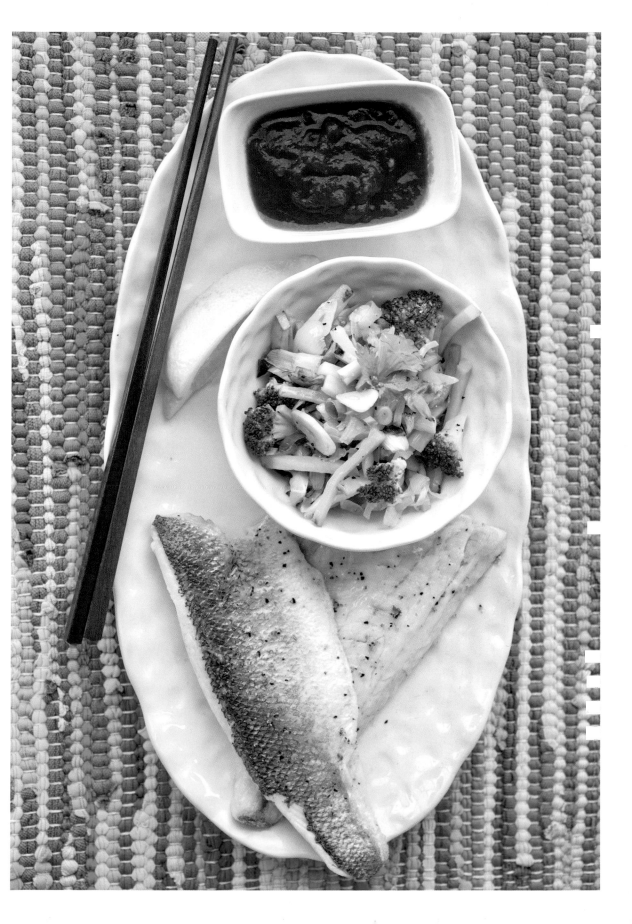

Galangal red curry with fish sauce

I made this recipe one day while in a mad rush and it turned out well—the spices give it a great taste. It is slightly higher in calories and carbohydrates than some of the others, so match it with a low carb and low calorie breakfast and lunch.

SERVES **4**

500 g cabbage
150 g/1 green pepper
150 g/1 red pepper
300 g/1 big leek
400 g broccoli
2 garlic cloves
light spray oil
4 pieces of galangal
6 kaffir lime leaves
2 tsp soy sauce

2 tbsp fish sauce
400 g chicken
1 tsp Thai red curry paste
juice of 1 lime
1 tbsp turmeric
1 cube vegetable or chicken stock in
    300 ml boiling water
Option: add 1–2 tsp low calorie sweetener
    if you wish to sweeten the dish

HOW TO PREPARE:

1 Wash the vegetables.

2 Cut cabbage, green and red pepper in thin strips. Cut leeks down the centre and then in half rounds. Cut broccoli in florets. Crush garlic.

3 Spray a wok with light spray oil and heat. Add galangal and kaffir lime leaves, soy sauce and fish sauce.

4 Cut chicken in strips and add to wok, along with curry paste and lime juice.

5 Add turmeric to wok and stir well.

6 Start with the cabbage, which takes longest to cook. Close lid and add boiling water from the kettle.

7 Add leeks to wok and cover with lid to allow steam to build up and vegetables to cook. However, remove lid to allow excess water to evaporate.

8 Melt vegetable stock in 300 ml of boiling water from kettle and add to the stir-fry mixture if contents are sticking to wok.

9 After 5 minutes add broccoli, peppers and garlic to wok and stir.

10 Place the lid over your stir-fry for 5 minutes and let simmer until vegetables are crunchy and chicken is cooked thoroughly.

11 Remove galangal and lime leaves and serve.

APPROXIMATELY **325** KCAL, 17.6 G CARBOHYDRATE PER SERVING

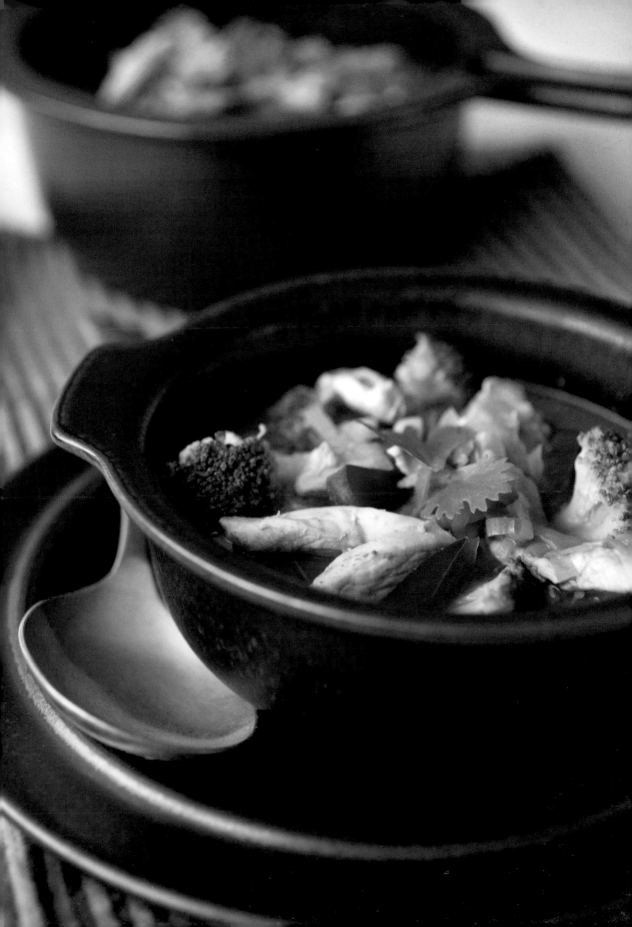

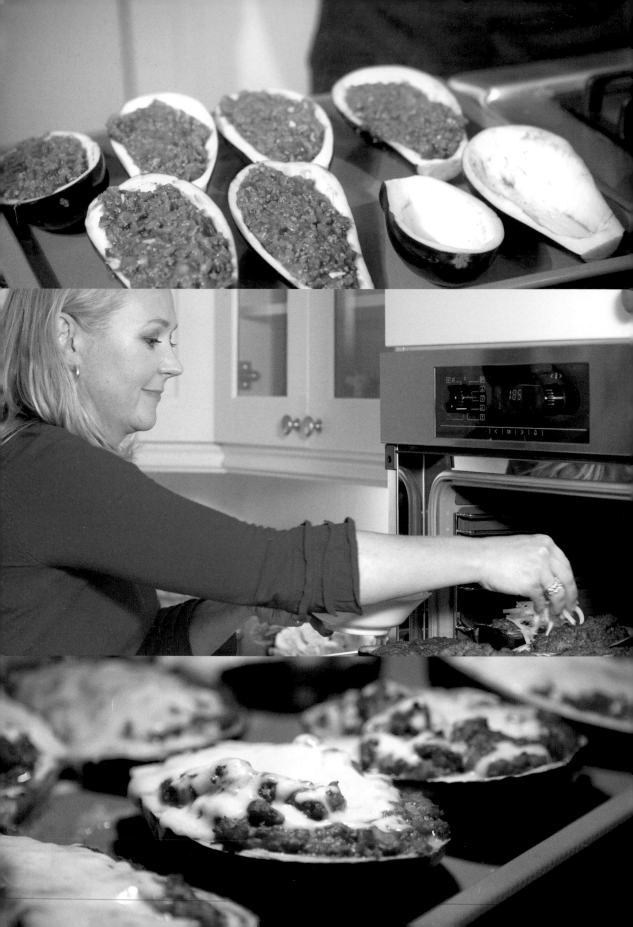

Aubergines stuffed with meat ratatouille

This is a delicious recipe—a little bit of work but worth the effort. This would not seem out of place at a dinner party as a starter and can be served with a fresh garden salad.

SERVES 4

1.4 kg/4–6 aubergines
300 g/3 leeks
light spray oil
6 garlic cloves, crushed
400 g lean minced meat
800 g/2 (400 g) cans of whole peeled
  tomatoes

1 beef stock cube
black pepper
4 tsp low calorie sweetener
250 g light mozzarella cheese, grated

tinfoil

HOW TO PREPARE:

1 Preheat the oven to 200 °C. Wash and cut aubergines in half lengthways. Using a serrated (sharp) knife, cut out the central flesh of the aubergine halves, leaving a 1 cm (½ inch) shell. Cut the flesh into 1 cm chunks.

2 Wash and cut leeks in half rounds.

3 Spray a non-stick pan with oil and heat. Add leeks and garlic and gently fry for 2 minutes until soft.

4 Add the minced meat and fry on a high heat until the meat is browned.

5 Next add the aubergine chunks, whole peeled tomatoes, stock cube and pepper and stir together.

6 Sprinkle the sweetener and stir. Simmer with the lid off over moderate heat until excess liquid has evaporated and you have a rich thick sauce.

7 Lightly spray your oven dish on which you are going to place the aubergine halves. Pile the vegetable meat filling inside the aubergines. Place in the oven, cover with tinfoil and bake for 20–40 minutes until cooked depending on your oven and the size of the aubergines.

8 Arrange the mozzarella over the filling for the last 5 minutes of cooking and continue cooking uncovered. Remove from oven and serve.

NOTE: This can be used as a family meal or alternatively you can make this dish in bulk and freeze some portions for future use. Two halves is a portion.

APPROXIMATELY **3 1 7** KCAL, 21.1 G CARBOHYDRATE PER SERVING

Rhubarb and jelly

SERVES 4

500 g rhubarb
5 tbsp low calorie sweetener
500 ml water
1 sachet of gelatine (that sets 500 ml of liquid depending on the brand you use)

4 glass bowls or cocktail glasses (heat proof or use a mug)

HOW TO PREPARE:

1 Wash and chop rhubarb.
2 Place rhubarb in a pot and cover with cold water.
3 Bring to boil.
4 Simmer for 5 minutes or until pulp is produced.
5 Take off the heat and stir in sweetener and gelatine. Ensure it is mixed well.
6 Pour mixture into cocktail glasses. I have served mine here in a glass that is suitable for hot mulled wine. Otherwise allow mixture to cool before pouring into glass.
7 Option: Place pieces of raw rhubarb at the bottom of the glass before adding in the mixture for nicer presentation.
8 Place in the fridge until set.

APPROXIMATELY 10 KCAL PER SERVING

Lemon surprise

SERVES 1

1 lemon
250 ml water
125 ml low calorie sweetener
juice of 2–3 lemons (125 ml lemon juice)
125 ml Diet 7up
few strips of lemon zest for garnish

HOW TO PREPARE:
1   Wash the lemon very well. Grate a few strips of lemon
    zest to garnish and set aside. Peel the rest of the lemon
    and dice finely. In a saucepan stir together the diced
    lemon peel, water and low calorie sweetener. Bring to
    boil, reduce heat and simmer for a few minutes. Remove
    from heat and allow to cool.
2   In a bowl stir together the cooled lemon syrup with the
    peel, freshly squeezed lemon juice and Diet 7up. Pour
    into an ice-cream maker, and freeze according to
    manufacturer's instructions.
3   Garnish each serving with a twist of lemon peel.

If you do not have an ice-cream maker, you may freeze it in
a tall canister. Freeze for 1½ hours. Remove and stir with a
whisk. Return to the freezer and stir once every hour for
about 4 hours. The more times you stir, the more air will be
incorporated, resulting in a lighter product.

APPROXIMATELY 22 KCAL PER SERVING

Chapter 7:
Dietary factors in health

WHAT YOU EAT will have a huge impact on your general health. It's important to ensure you eat a balanced diet. In this chapter I will outline the importance of specific elements in the diet as well as the effects of high cholesterol. If your body is not working as well as it should, there are a number of blood tests you can have done to find out the cause, so I will outline these. Diabetes is a huge problem in Ireland and diet can affect its onset and treatment. I will describe this.

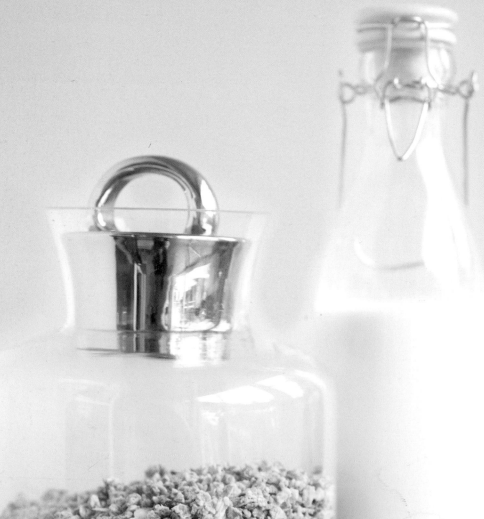

Calcium

Calcium is needed to build and maintain bone strength and it is also important for nerve-signal transmission. The recommended daily amount (RDA) of calcium for children aged 1–10 years is 800 mg. Adults require 1,000 mg per day up to 50 years of age while teenagers, and pregnant and breastfeeding women and adults over 50 years need 1,200 mg per day.

If these quantities are not met, calcium is reabsorbed from the bone, creating weakening of the bone mass and locally reducing the strength. This is better known as osteoporosis or brittle bone disease, which causes bones to break or fracture easily. It is estimated that one in three women and one in 12 men over the age of 55 years will suffer from osteoporosis in their lifetime.

Risk factors for osteoporosis, such as age, being female and having a family history of the illness, cannot be changed. However, lifestyle risk factors that can be changed include:

- **Ensuring you have a balanced daily diet and that you have a sufficient calcium intake.**

- **Giving up smoking.**

- **Taking regular exercise outdoors. Weight-bearing exercises like walking or jogging are excellent.**

- **Drinking no more than 2 units of alcohol a day if you are a woman and no more than 3 units if you are a man.**

- **Drinking no more than 2–3 cups of strong coffee a day.**

CALCIUM SOURCES

Dairy products such as milk, cheese and yoghurt are the most commonly known source of calcium. There is 119 mg of calcium in 100 ml of milk. While dairy is a rich source of calcium, it is a mineral that is also present in other food groups such as leafy green vegetables and fish. For example, 100 g of tinned salmon has 214 mg of calcium and a few florets (100 g) of broccoli contain 56 mg. Some foods that can also contribute to total intake include calcium-fortified cereals, soya milk, etc.

Therefore it is still possible to get adequate calcium even if following a dairy-free diet by choosing alternative food groups that are calcium-rich.

Vitamin D

Unfortunately, only 10 per cent of calcium taken into the body is absorbed and there are other substances that can affect calcium absorption. Vitamin D is of fundamental importance for the absorption process. Vitamin D is actually not a vitamin but a hormone. Our bodies make the 'sunshine' vitamin through the action of ultraviolet light and heat on the skin creating the conversion of provitamin D to vitamin D. We can also get sufficient vitamin D through dietary choices. Oily fish such as herring, mackerel, salmon and trout are good sources. However, since these foods are not eaten frequently, it is difficult to achieve the recommended levels through diet alone. Cod liver oil or vitamin D fortified foods, such as some milks, yogurts and cereals, are useful alternative sources. The RDA for vitamin D is 7.5 ug for adults, 10 ug (equivalent to 400 IU) for children and the over-70s.

Cholesterol

'High cholesterol' is the worrying term. Governments throughout the world are battling with increasing medical expenses and different solutions are being sought on how to reduce costs. High cholesterol, Type 2 diabetes and high blood pressure medications are some of the biggest expenses health providers are facing today. Statin medication is known to have one of the highest ingredient costs under the Community Drugs Scheme in Ireland.

Most of these patients could be treated with the right lifestyle modification and diet advice. Prevention of a disease is substantially less expensive in the long run and many of the most costly (in human and financial terms) chronic diseases could be prevented and treated with lifestyle changes.

When a doctor discovers high cholesterol levels in a patient, they give the patient a list of foods to avoid and foods to include in their diet in order to lower cholesterol. The aim is to reduce calories from saturated fats to <10 per cent and to have plenty of gel-forming fibre, and exercise. If, after three months, cholesterol has not dropped to acceptable levels with the dietary approach, the patient is prescribed statin medication and a diagnosis of familial hypercholesterolemia is made. These statins are very effective in reducing the cholesterol levels and once a patient is on this medication, they usually stay on it for life.

This gets one risk factor under control but has not solved the problem—and we still don't know all the long-term side effects of these medications. Just think, if 60 per cent of your brain is fat, what will these statins do to it? Most of the patients diagnosed with high cholesterol are also overweight or obese. Although the doctor may advise them to lose weight, eat less and exercise more, this task is left up to the patient. In most cases the patient will fail because losing weight requires a sustainable lifestyle change. This is difficult to put into action without plenty of specific advice and support. If you don't know what you are eating and how it affects your body, how can you be expected to make positive changes to your diet?

There are two main types of cholesterol in our body that changes in relation to dietary intake and exercise: LDL and HDL cholesterol. LDL cholesterol (the bad cholesterol) is transported through the blood to the body's tissues. If the levels are too high, the build-up on the inside of the arteries could result in a heart attack or stroke. The second type of cholesterol, HDL, is the opposite of LDL in function. HDL is cholesterol that is transported from organs and tissues to be used or eliminated, so a high HDL level in the blood is considered protective against heart disease and stroke.

For years it was thought that only a high fat intake would influence our cholesterol levels, but it now appears that the types of carbohydrates we choose also play a significant role. From studies on diabetes, it has been found that even in cases where diet is low in fat, the subjects still had high cholesterol. It is becoming clear that high sugar levels or a high glycaemic diet affects blood cholesterol levels through the mechanism of continuous high circulating insulin levels. There are plenty of slim people in the world who have high cholesterol levels. A typical example would be a person who has a diet comprising a large proportion of processed carbohydrates but not enough fruit and vegetables. They are not overeating, but they do not have an overall balanced diet, in my opinion.

If high cholesterol is a problem, then the first approach should be to follow a low glycaemic diet plan. But you should also watch the types of fats you eat to maintain overall health (see Chapter 9).

Glucose

Fasting blood glucose is measured to diagnose diabetes. Type 2 diabetes, which is closely linked to obesity, usually develops silently over several years without showing any symptoms until the day when the first complication presents itself. This could be a mild form of heart attack or only a slight discomfort during increased activity, and angina is diagnosed.

It is estimated that it takes around seven years between the onset of Type 2 diabetes and the diagnosis of this common disease. As the disease develops, it follows a gradual process of increasing blood glucose, from impaired glucose tolerance (IGT), to impaired fasting glucose (IFG) and eventually diabetes. These pre-diabetes conditions were not previously considered dangerous but as our knowledge has increased, we now know that if we are able to identify this early stage of the disease, we can reverse the disease process through lifestyle changes.

As the person has no symptoms, the only way to screen is through fasting blood sample.

When an abnormal fasting glucose result is found, the next step should be a test called the oral glucose tolerance test. Only if this test shows fasting glucose levels above the norm can a diagnosis of diabetes be made. Diabetes should not be diagnosed based on one single abnormal blood glucose value.

Blood tests

Blood tests are usually taken by a General Practitioner (GP) to discover underlying causes for a particular complaint that a patient presents. The general opinion of the medical profession has been that it is unnecessary to start screening for disease in people without specific complaints. However, I feel that it is important to identify any medical risk factors and to exclude a possible medical cause for weight gain.

When you are young, your body can still handle extra weight but with time the wear and tear will take its toll. However, for morbidly obese people (BMI over 40), the symptoms appear rapidly and the consequences can be fatal. Even being slightly overweight causes your body to come under attack and have to deal with extra pressure.

The most important reasons for getting your blood tested are as follows:

- **To screen for general health status—this is done with a full blood count.**
- **To screen for common risk factors like cholesterol and diabetes.**
- **To discover possible metabolic reasons for weight gain like underactive thyroid or Cushing's syndrome (a very uncommon and rare hormonal disorder).**
- **To discover possible nutritional deficiencies like low iron, low B12 or low folic acid.**
- **To discover possible common genetic diseases like haemochromatosis (excessive iron absorption).**

Overweight—and more commonly obese—people generally suffer from low energy levels, joint and bone pains, sleeping problems, breathing difficulties, digestive complaints, infertility and many more everyday medical problems. These are usually weight related but the blood test will help to identify if there are any other reasons for these symptoms.

It is important to have your bloods taken after 14 hours of fasting (you can drink only water for 14 hours prior to the test) so that your sugar levels and body functions are not being influenced by your last meal or night out on the town.

Your GP will advise you before the bloods are taken.

I have seen a number of cases of undiagnosed medical conditions because patients did not have their bloods tested regularly. Blood tests will indicate, amongst others, underactive thyroid or anaemia—issues that should be identified before commencing a diet. It is important to establish that you are healthy before dieting.

SO, WHAT CAN A BLOOD TEST TELL US?

The full blood count (FBC) comprises the red blood cell count (RBC), haemoglobin (Hb), white blood count (WBC) and platelets count (PLTS).

Red blood cells are responsible for delivering oxygen throughout the body. Haemoglobin is the protein in them that makes this exchange possible. If the haemoglobin concentration is less than 12.0 g/dl, this is called anaemia and the oxygen delivery is deficient, resulting in tiredness. This can mainly be caused by deficiencies in iron, B12 and folate.

The white blood cells are responsible for defending the body against infection. The most common reason for the white blood count being high is bacterial infection. Decrease is usually due to viral infection.

Platelets are important to help stop bleeding. Decrease can be due to several reasons but severe infection is a common cause.

There are a number of other blood tests that can be done.

Liver Function Tests (LFT): Liver enzymes (AST, ALT and GGT) will increase in any condition involving destruction of the liver cells (hepatocytes). The most common cause of an increase is high alcohol consumption. However, OW (overweight) people, who would typically have high cholesterol, will find that their liver has small deposits of fat—this is called fatty liver disease. In my clinics I see huge improvements in liver function tests and fatty deposits with even modest weight loss. The use of painkillers, together with fatty liver, is the most common cause of a raise in liver function test results.

Thyroid function: The thyroid affects almost everything in our body. Low energy levels, high cholesterol, weight gain and depression are some of the main symptoms of an underactive thyroid. In my experience, most OW people have at least one of the symptoms indicating the malfunctioning of this organ but this is usually due to excess weight rather than thyroid dysfunction.

Glucose—fasting glucose: This is mainly taken to exclude diabetes. Type 2 diabetes, which is closely linked to obesity, usually develops silently over several years without showing any symptoms until the day when the first complication shows. (See the section on diabetes on p.77.)

Glucose tolerance test: This is used to confirm the diagnosis of Type 2 diabetes. The test measures the glucose concentration in the blood 2 hours after consuming 75 g of soluble glucose. A reading of over 11.1 mmol/L indicates the presence of Type 2 diabetes.

Full fasting lipid profile: Lipid means fat. This test gives results for Low Density Lipoprotein (LDL), High Density Lipoprotein (HDL) and Triglycerides. LDL is 'bad' cholesterol. HDL is 'good' cholesterol and protects you against cardiovascular disease. If your HDL level is high, it is actually a negative risk factor and balances out other heart disease risk factors. Triglycerides are fats that are transported to tissues for energy or they are stored as fat. Your total cholesterol level should be under 5 mmol/L. LDL should be under 2.6 mmol/L and HDL should be over 1.1 mmol/L for men and over 1.3 mmol/L for women. Triglycerides should be under 1.7 mmol/L. Raised Triglycerides can be the first sign of Type 2 diabetes, apparent even before raised blood glucose levels are detected.

Kidney Function Test: This is one of the most commonly performed blood tests to check that kidneys are working properly. Urea and creatinine are waste products formed from the breakdown of protein and muscle respectively, and are usually excreted in urine. High blood level indicates that the kidneys are not working properly. Creatinine is usually a more accurate marker of kidney function than urea. A high urea level in blood can also indicate that you are dehydrated. This happens often when people don't drink water before a fasting blood sample is taken. Two of the most common causes of kidney disease are diabetes and high blood pressure, both of which are associated with being overweight and obese. Diabetic nephropathy (damage to the kidney) is a leading cause of end-stage renal failure. High blood glucose levels can cause damage to the nephrons, causing diabetic kidney disease. Controlling glucose levels can delay or prevent kidney damage. High blood pressure can damage the small blood vessels in the kidneys, inhibiting the blood vessels to filter waste from the blood efficiently.

B12 and folate: With iron, these three are necessary ingredients to make haemoglobin. If B12 and folate are deficient, this will result in anaemia. Vegetarians are at risk of running their B12 reserves low because this vitamin is nonexistent in vegetables. Although B12 deficiency can be caused by a poor diet, it can also be down to poor absorption in the body. In this case no amount of dietary B12 will reverse the problem and B12 injections will need to be administered.

Ferritin: This is a measure of iron stores. Almost a third of women aged 18 to 50 years have inadequate iron stores, exposing them to increased risk of iron deficiency or anaemia. This is typically due to heavy periods and an unbalanced diet. Excess iron absorption (haemochromatosis) will result in iron loading of the liver, heart, pancreas, joints and pituitary. This is a common inherited disorder in some countries (Ireland, for example) but the cure is simple if diagnosed early. If left untreated, haemochromatosis can lead to hardening of the liver. It has been found that slightly raised iron levels in the overweight or obese can indicate generalised inflammation of the body. This can be improved by weight loss.

Bilirubin: This is a brownish-yellow waste substance found in bile. It is produced when the liver breaks down old red blood cells and is removed from the body through the stool (faeces). Jaundice can occur when bilirubin levels are high. Symptoms include yellowing of the whites of the eyes and skin. Jaundice may be caused by liver disease, blood disorders such as haemolytic and pernicious anaemia, and blockage of the bile ducts that allow bile to pass from the liver to the small intestine.

Syndrome X

If you have had a fasting blood screen done by your GP and have your other physical measurements—visceral/central fat, blood pressure—you can now assess how many risk factors you carry for Syndrome X, also called metabolic syndrome. A person with any three of the following five conditions would be classified as having Syndrome X:

- **Waist circumference (central obesity): women >92 cm (36 inches), men >102 cm (40 inches)**
- **Elevated fasting blood Triglycerides >1.7 mmol/L**
- **Low levels of HDL cholesterol: women <1.3 mmol/L, men <1.1 mmol/L**
- **High blood pressure or BP >135/85**
- **Diabetes or fasting glucose >6 mmol/L**

The term Syndrome X, or metabolic syndrome, is a mild form of diabetes or a condition that creates similar consequences. However, the main difference is that with Syndrome X the body produces excess insulin that compensates and suppresses the typical indicators used to identify diabetes. It is very likely that a person suffering from Syndrome X will develop full-blown Type 2 diabetes.

Fortunately, research has shown that within 11 weeks of a lifestyle change some of the damage done to the arteries in the heart and brain will start reversing. So it's never too late to begin.

Diabetes

According to WHO, approximately 220 million people suffer from diabetes worldwide. It is estimated that in 2011 there were about 180,000 people, of all age groups, with diabetes in Ireland (Type 1 and Type 2 populations combined). On top of this there were up to 50,000 people who have undiagnosed Type 2 diabetes. More worryingly, according to Diabetes Ireland, there are at least a further 130,000 people in Ireland who have pre-diabetes (borderline Type 2 diabetes), half of whom will develop Type 2 diabetes in the next five years unless they make lifestyle changes. However, endocrinologists I have dealt with believe that the number of borderline Type 2 cases is more likely to be in the region of 250,000–350,000.

There are two types of diabetes:

1 Type 1 diabetes (insulin-dependent diabetes) is a chronic condition, which requires insulin injections. The condition develops when an autoimmune reaction causes the pancreas to stop producing insulin. When the pancreas does not produce insulin, sugar can't be used by cells. Symptoms of Type 1 diabetes are extreme thirst, frequent urination, sugar in the urine, an acetone-like smell around the body, fatigue, and substantial weight loss over a short period of time. Type 1 diabetes is usually diagnosed before the age of 40.

2 Type 2 diabetes is more common and accounts for over 90 per cent of all diabetes cases around the world. It is largely the result of excess body weight. People with this type of diabetes produce too little insulin or the insulin they produce cannot work properly because their body has become resistant to insulin. Almost every one of us could develop Type 2 diabetes if we gain enough weight. This form is more common in people over 40 years of age but it is becoming much more common in young people as childhood obesity is now on the increase. Obese people and people who have a relative already suffering from this disease are more likely to be affected. Approximately 90 per cent of patients with Type 2 diabetes are obese. Half of the cases of Type 2 diabetes are without symptoms and can only be discovered with testing sugar (glucose) in the urine or blood.

You are at high risk of developing Type 2 diabetes if:

- **You are over 40.**

- **You are overweight.**

- **You have a family history of Type 2 diabetes.**

Type 2 diabetes is a progressive disease and it has been estimated that it begins to develop approximately seven years before it is diagnosed. This means that unknown high blood sugar levels are silently causing damage to the body. At diagnosis a patient can often present with one or all of the following symptoms: bad eyesight, pains in feet and hands, extreme tiredness, unnatural thirst, ulcers on the legs. In advanced cases, the first symptom can be a heart attack or stroke.

Over time, diabetes can damage the heart, blood vessels, eyes, kidneys and nerves through:

- Heart disease and stroke: 50 per cent of people with diabetes die of cardiovascular disease.

- Retinopathy: This results from accumulated damage to the small blood vessels in the retina and is a common cause of blindness. After 15 years of diabetes, approximately 2 per cent of people become blind, and about 10 per cent develop severe visual impairment.

- Kidney failure: This results in 10–20 per cent of diabetic-related deaths.

- Neuropathy: This is damage to the nerves as a result of diabetes, and affects up to 50 per cent of people with diabetes. Although many different problems can occur as a result of diabetic neuropathy, common symptoms are tingling, pain, numbness, or weakness in the feet and hands. It can lead to foot ulcers and limb amputation, especially when combined with poor circulation.

The overall risk of death for people with diabetes is at least double the risk of their peers without diabetes.

TREATMENT

Type 1 diabetes has to be treated with insulin injections. However, with specific dietary changes, medication can be significantly reduced. On the other hand, Type 2 diabetes can be reversed with simple lifestyle measures. To help prevent Type 2 diabetes and its complications, you should:

- Watch your weight: Achieving and maintaining a healthy body weight is essential in the prevention and treatment of diabetes, i.e. maintain a BMI of 20–25.

- Exercise: At least 30 minutes of regular, moderate-intensity activity on most days. More activity is required for weight control.

- Eat a healthy balanced diet.

VLCDS IN TREATMENT OF DIABETES

Although traditionally it is thought that a healthy eating plan is the best course of action for diabetes treatment, new research carried out by Diabetes UK found that following a Very Low Calorie Diet (VLCD) is effective in reversing Type 2 diabetes.

The study found that a simple eight-week intensive diet followed by a healthy eating plan could do away with the need for years of expensive medication.

Patients were put on a strict diet of just 600 calories a day, consisting of slimming shakes, non-starchy vegetables, tea and zero-calorie drinks. After just one week, early morning blood sugar levels had returned to normal, and after two months the fat in the pancreas had returned to normal and the pancreas was producing insulin normally. After three months the patients were reviewed. All of them had resumed normal eating with advice on portion control and healthy foods. Seven out of the 11 people remained free of diabetes.

This is major news and could revolutionise the way people with Type 2 diabetes are treated. This study confirms findings that I have seen first-hand with numerous patients who have Type 2 diabetes at my clinics. I have witnessed drastic improvements in overall glucose levels (HbA1c levels) in a matter of weeks after following our diet plans. I have devised Phase 1 in this book to be a VLCD. However, it should not be followed for more than 10 days. Anyone with a medical condition and especially diabetics should always follow this type of diet under medical supervision.

ALCOHOL

There is conflicting evidence regarding alcohol recommendations for people with diabetes. The Nutrition Subcommittee of the Diabetes Care Advisory Committee of Diabetes UK 2003 as well as Diabetes Federation of Ireland gives the same recommendations for people with diabetes as the rest of the population, i.e. 14 units per week for women and 21 units per week for men, and 1–2 alcohol-free days. However, further research carried out by the nutrition study group of the European Association for the Study of Diabetes 2004 recommends a moderate use of alcohol—up to 1 unit (10 g) per day for women and 2 units (20 g) per day for men. The American Diabetes Association 2007 also recommends that daily alcohol intake should be limited to a moderate amount, i.e. 1.5 units (15 g) alcohol per day for women and 2 units (30 g) alcohol per day for men. A unit is half a pint of beer, 1 small (100 ml) glass of wine or 1 bottle of alcopop (See pp. 85–7.)

Drinking alcohol is generally not a good idea if you are diabetic.

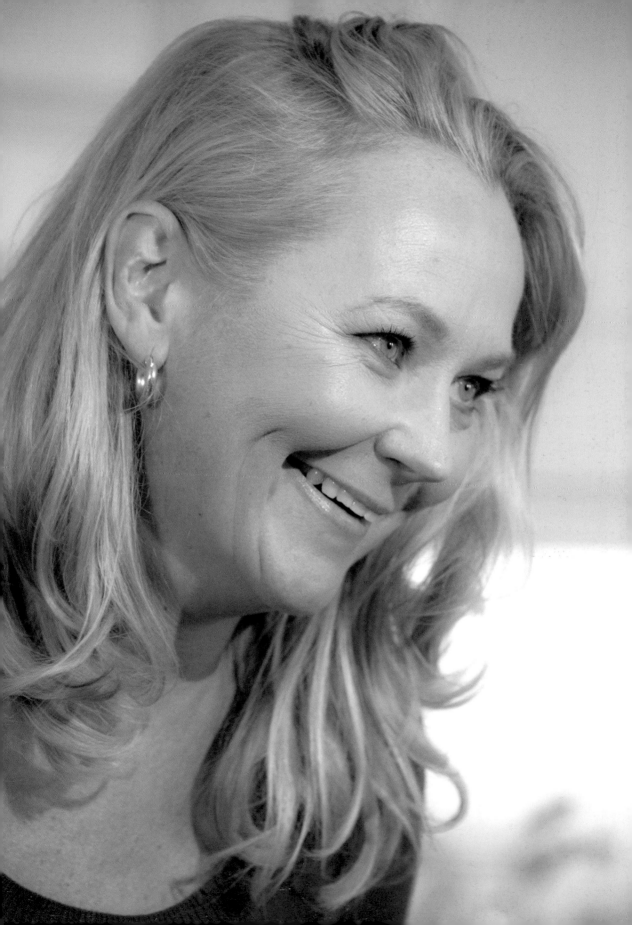

Chapter 8:
Phase 2—
1,200 kcal diet

PHASE 2 IS more nutritionally balanced than Phase 1 due to the re-introduction of complex carbohydrates. You are no longer in ketosis. However, as this diet is based on 1,200 kcal per day, you will still be in an energy deficit of approximately 800 kcal/day for women and 1,300 kcal/day for men from your diet alone. Therefore the body will still be forced to draw the extra energy from your fat stores.

On this phase a woman will lose approximately 1–1.5 kg (2.2–3.3 lb) per week—depending on size and activity levels. Men can expect to achieve slightly higher results at 1.5–2.5 kg (3.3–5.5 lb) per week—again depending on size and activity levels. This phase also re-introduces you gradually to a balanced diet while incorporating behaviour modification in the practice of portion control, increased food choice and more food variety. This diet is still high in protein and vegetables, but includes some dairy and complex carbohydrates as well.

Choosing carbohydrate foods that provide a slow release of energy helps to maintain stable blood sugar levels and prevent cravings. Confectionery and sweets should still be avoided. This plan is still low calorie but based on healthy eating guidelines. Weight loss will be slower on this plan than on Phase 1. Phase 2 also requires portion control to ensure calories are kept low. However, there is more food choice, making the diet more interesting.

Phase 2 is recommended as a follow-on diet for people who have completed Phase 1 and now have a BMI of 30. Alternatively, it can be a first phase option for people who have a BMI in this range. This phase is also suitable for anyone who wishes to learn how to change their eating habits to ensure long-term success while continuing to lose weight.

Side effects

You may experience some hunger on the plan as you are out of ketosis, but this should be minimum if you have my filler soup.

Exercise

Exercise is encouraged in this phase to aid weight loss. Also, as exercise is essential in the weight-maintenance stage, now is a great time to start introducing it into your lifestyle so that it becomes a regular habit. Gentle regular exercise such as walking or swimming is a good way to start. In addition, regular activity will help you to sleep better, which is important for your overall health.

The importance of sleep

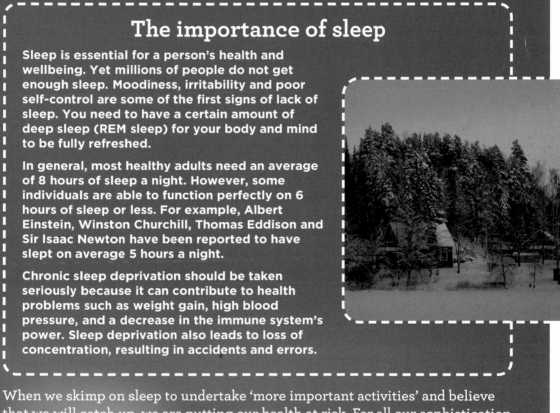

Sleep is essential for a person's health and wellbeing. Yet millions of people do not get enough sleep. Moodiness, irritability and poor self-control are some of the first signs of lack of sleep. You need to have a certain amount of deep sleep (REM sleep) for your body and mind to be fully refreshed.

In general, most healthy adults need an average of 8 hours of sleep a night. However, some individuals are able to function perfectly on 6 hours of sleep or less. For example, Albert Einstein, Winston Churchill, Thomas Eddison and Sir Isaac Newton have been reported to have slept on average 5 hours a night.

Chronic sleep deprivation should be taken seriously because it can contribute to health problems such as weight gain, high blood pressure, and a decrease in the immune system's power. Sleep deprivation also leads to loss of concentration, resulting in accidents and errors.

When we skimp on sleep to undertake 'more important activities' and believe that we will catch up, we are putting our health at risk. For all our sophistication and civilised ways of living, we must remember that our brain and body are governed by biological functions and needs. Sleep plays a huge part in the way our bodies function—so much so, in fact, that if we are totally deprived of sleep for an extended period of time, we will die.

So what has this got to do with weight loss?

Recent research indicates that a good sleeping pattern is a fundamental part of any weight-loss programme. When you are tired, your blood sugar levels can drop, making you crave high energy foods.

Feeling tired can also make you feel lazy. You will be less inclined to cook a healthy meal and more inclined to choose a convenience food or easy-to-make meal that is usually higher in fat and calories.

Hormonal changes that occur as a result of sleep deprivation can also affect your weight. Ghrelin, a hormone responsible for the feeling of hunger, is increased when a person is tired, which therefore means you will have a bigger appetite. Simultaneously, leptin, a hormone responsible for the feeling of satiety and which tells the brain when it is time to stop eating, is reduced when you are tired, further enhancing the likelihood of overeating. The combined effect of these hormonal changes can sabotage your diet attempts.

TIPS TO COMBAT COMMON SLEEP PROBLEMS:
- **Keep a regular sleep/wake schedule.**
- **Don't drink caffeine 4 to 6 hours before bedtime and minimise daytime consumption.**
- **Don't smoke, especially near bedtime or if you wake in the night.**
- **Avoid alcohol, heavy meals and high energy foods (e.g. chocolate) before sleep.**
- **Take regular exercise.**
- **Sleep in an environment that is quiet, dark and a comfortable temperature.**

Relaxation just before bed is beneficial when you wish to wind down. It is a natural sleep aid that helps calm your mind so you fall asleep. Relaxation also helps you to fall asleep in a positive frame of mind, which can result in a more peaceful sleep.

In Finland we say that sleeping is like putting money in the bank.

Sleep apnoea

Sleep apnoea is a sleep disorder where the sufferer frequently stops breathing during their sleep. According to the Irish Sleep Apnoea Trust, breathing can stop repeatedly for 10 seconds and longer in extreme cases.

Sleep apnoea can result in a reduction in short-term memory, and disruption to social and family life. The condition usually goes undiagnosed, with only one in four people with obstructive sleep apnoea diagnosed with the condition. Left untreated, it can increase the risk of high blood pressure, heart attack, stroke, obesity and Type 2 diabetes. Somewhere in the region of 95,000–105,000 people in Ireland actually suffer from the disorder.

Eating out

Lean meat or fish served with salad or vegetables are the best options. You can choose from a whole variety of 'above' and 'below' ground vegetables but beware of calorie-laden creamy sauces and salad dressings. It would be better to avoid carbohydrates to keep overall calories low, although a very small portion of rice or pasta would be acceptable. You can now have one glass of wine (2 units) if you wish. Dessert should still be avoided.

Alcohol

Alcohol may be included in small amounts, such as the odd glass of wine or 1–2 spirits a week on Phase 2. This can be beneficial from a social point of view and it also encourages dietary compliance from people who find it hard to follow plans that completely eliminate alcohol. However, alcohol does contain calories and if the quantities are not kept to a minimum, it may raise your total daily calorie intake significantly. Also, as alcohol lowers blood sugar levels, you may experience a craving for carbohydrates, 'the munchies'. These cravings are difficult to ignore and will jeopardise your diet success. So remember, keep alcohol to a minimum and try to save it for special occasions. Reducing alcohol has many health benefits, not only good for your waistline.

Alcohol: the facts

Alcohol can have some beneficial effects on our health—but unfortunately only in small quantities!

Up to 2 units of alcohol a day (women) or 3 units (men) is known to be beneficial, but above these quantities, your health will suffer.

When assessing a person's risk factors, we used to ask 'How many units of alcohol do you drink in one week?' This question was actually misleading and nowadays the question asked is 'How many units do you drink per day?' The reason is simply that you cannot save up your units and consume them in one night. More than 5 units a day is considered binge drinking.

If you want to add years, health and quality to the rest of your life, then you need to learn some self-discipline and enforce moderation. We need to respect alcohol as a potential killer if used excessively. Every time you exceed your recommended units, you need to be aware that you are damaging your liver.

The first organ to suffer when alcohol enters your body is your mouth, and your tongue in particular! (This has been highlighted by the fact that tongue cancer is on the increase, and is made worse by smoking.) Excessive consumption of alcohol can cause irritation and inflammation of the stomach, leading to nausea and vomiting. Once alcohol has been absorbed from the stomach and small intestine, it is taken to the liver—the main detox organ in the body. This organ is then put under tremendous pressure to break the alcohol down and remove it from the body. A healthy liver is the major fat-burning organ in the body—it pumps excessive fat out of the body through the bile into the small intestine. It detoxifies, and controls the metabolism of fat. If the liver is kept too busy detoxifying the alcohol, it will inhibit its ability to metabolise the fat.

If the alcohol intake has been excessive for a long period, it is very likely to show up in the blood results in the form of high GGT (liver transaminase levels (see p75). So, excessive alcohol intake cannot be hidden from your doctor. Excessive alcohol also affects facial appearance and skin.

At the end of the day that longing for a glass of wine is 'learnt behaviour'. In the same way you learn to have it every evening, you can also learn not to have it! To help you manage your alcohol intake, you need to understand what a 'unit' of alcohol is!

ALCOHOL UNIT

A unit of alcohol is 10 ml or 10 g of pure alcohol (ethanol).

Simply saying that a unit of alcohol is a small (100 ml) glass of wine or a half pint of beer is very misleading because it does not take into consideration the huge differences in strengths and measures of wines, beers and spirits.

The number of units of alcohol in a drink depends on:

• How strong it is
• The volume of the drink

The number of units of alcohol can be determined by multiplying the volume of the drink (in litres) by its percentage alcohol (by volume) (ABV).

A 500 ml can of beer at 4.3 per cent ABV contains:

0.5 x 4.3 = 2.15 units of alcohol

On average a bottle of wine (750 ml) at 13 per cent contains 10 units of alcohol.

(0.75 x 13 = 9.8)

A few examples:

• A small 100 ml glass of wine at 9 per cent is 1 unit.
• A large glass (250 ml) contains 3.0 units.
• A 35.5 ml pub measure of vodka or whiskey at 40 per cent is 1.5 units in Ireland.
• A small glass (50 ml) of sherry, fortified wine or cream liqueur (approximately 20 per cent ABV) contains about 1 unit.

CALORIES IN ALCOHOL

There are 7 calories per gram of alcohol. This is only second to fat, at 9 cal/g. A few examples are:

Pint of Fosters	193 kcal
Pint of draught Guinness	210 kcal
Pint of Heineken	227 kcal
Gin and tonic	120 kcal
Smirnoff Ice	228 kcal
Jack Daniels—single (25 ml)	64 kcal
White wine—dry (175 ml)	116 kcal
Smirnoff Red (20 ml)	44 kcal
Champagne (175 ml)	133 kcal
Martini (single—50 ml)	70 kcal

Meal options

Breakfast 250 kcal, Lunch 300 kcal, Dinner 500 kcal, Snacks 150 kcal

Breakfast
1 Breakfast muffins with café latte
2 Oaty smoothie
3 Peachy porridge
4 Buckwheat porridge (gluten free)
5 Granola with banana and yoghurt

Lunch
You could alternatively make a salad, depending on the calories, See the Salad section on p.201.
1 Low fat turkey and coleslaw wrap
2 Creamy salmon quiche
3 Niçoise salad
4 Leek and potato soup with a vegetable you do not like
5 Cockle pasta

Dinner
1 Puy lentil stew
2 Guinness casserole
3 Monkfish wrapped in bacon with stir-fried vegetables
4 Indian chicken with herbs and couscous
5 Grilled tuna steak with Italian peperonata
6 Madras lamb curry
7 Thai green turkey curry
8 Beef au vin à la Eva
You can also select meals from Phase 1.

Snacks

You can choose 3 of the 50 kcal snacks in the Phase 1 list, or 1 of the 150 kcal snacks from this list each day.

- 2 tbsp green lentil hummus spread (see p.208). Serve with half a wholegrain pitta bread (150 kcal)
- 2 rice cakes, 80 g low fat cottage cheese and cucumber slices (146 kcal)
- 1 medium apple (100 g) sliced and served with 40 g chopped reduced fat cheddar cheese (149 kcal)
- 30 g tortilla chips (approximately 12) with 2 tbsp salsa (152 kcal)
- 1 low fat yoghurt and 1 packet cheese strings (60 kcal)

Below: breakfast muffins

Breakfast recipes

Breakfast muffins with café latte

A patient of mine gave me the idea for this recipe, which has a lower calorie content than the average muffin. A muffin with a chocolate filling is easily 500 kcal but this one is only 250 kcal with a café latte.

MAKES **8**

150 g wholemeal flour
110 g unprocessed bran
100 g dried apricots, finely chopped
1 tsp bicarbonate of soda
1 tsp ground cinnamon
1 tsp ground nutmeg
1 egg, beaten
4 tbsp low calorie sweetener
2 tbsp hazelnut oil
1 tsp natural vanilla extract
185 ml full fat milk

Latte
100 ml water
200 ml low fat milk
1 tsp coffee (or to your taste)

HOW TO PREPARE:

1 Preheat oven to 200 °C.

2 Mix all the dry ingredients together, making sure the apricots are finely chopped. Try to use apricots that have a little moisture in them, e.g. Shamrock.

3 Combine the wet ingredients with the dry ingredients.

4 Place 8 muffin cases on a muffin tray and spoon the mixture into the cases.

5 Bake for 15 minutes or until skewer comes out clean.

6 Cool on a wire rack.

7 Serve with your own homemade latte. Make your coffee with hot water and hot milk.

APPROXIMATELY **250** KCAL FOR 1 MUFFIN AND 1 CAFÉ LATTE

Oaty smoothie

This is delicious. Oats are soluble fibre, known to help lower cholesterol. The smoothie is also dairy and soya free.

SERVES **2**

100 g banana (peeled weight)
75 g ready to eat dried prunes (4.3 g fibre)
40 g wholegrain rolled oats (porridge oats)
200 ml Rice dream milk

HOW TO PREPARE:

1 Peel and chop your banana.

2 Put all the ingredients into a blender and blend until smooth.

3 Serve in a glass.

4 This smoothie provides 3.4 g fibre per serving and is a good source of calcium and vitamins. It is suitable for those on vegetarian, dairy-free and soya-free diets.

APPROXIMATELY **230** KCAL PER SERVING

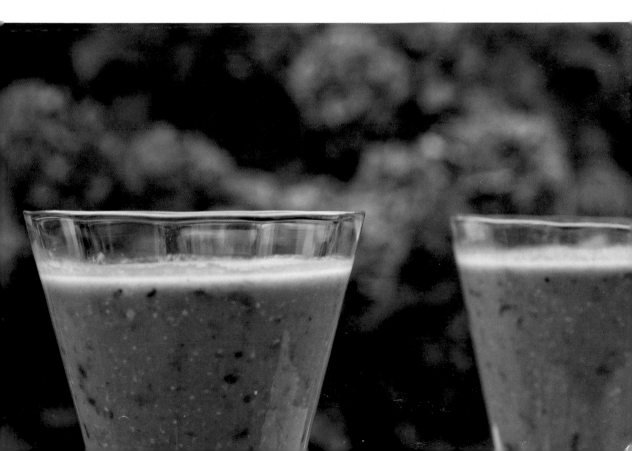

Peachy porridge

This is nice even if you don't have fresh fruit—it's easy to liquidise tinned peaches. They give a nice flavour to porridge.

SERVES **4**

160 g oats (40 g per person)
600 ml water
180 g/2 peaches cut in half

HOW TO PREPARE:

1   Start cooking oats with water.

2   While they cook, purée the peaches with a blender.

3   When oats are almost cooked, add peach purée. I find that the peach gives enough sweetness to the oats but if you prefer a sweeter version, add more low calorie sweetener.

Simple but healthy and delicious!

APPROXIMATELY **200** KCAL PER SERVING

Buckwheat porridge (gluten free)

Various studies have been done worldwide to show the benefits of buckwheat, including reducing blood cholesterol and blood pressure due to its bioflavonoid content.

SERVES **1**

40 g buckwheat flakes (available in health food shops)
250 ml water
100 g blueberries

HOW TO PREPARE:

1   Mix buckwheat with water and bring to boil. Reduce heat down to simmer and cook for 4 minutes, stirring frequently.

2   Stir in blueberries and serve.

APPROXIMATELY **190** KCAL PER SERVING
OPTION: Alternatively use only 50 g of blueberries, and use 200 ml water and 50 ml low-fat Supermilk to obtain a creamier consistency.

APPROXIMATELY **187** KCAL PER SERVING

Buckwheat is used as a grain although it is not one. You can also find products such as buckwheat noodles and crackers in the supermarket. Owing to its strong flavour, it is typically used only as part of the total flour content in baking.

Benefits of buckwheat:
- Naturally gluten free.
- Lower in carbohydrates, calories and fats than oats.
- Higher in protein than oats and similar in fibre content.
- Very versatile and can be used in cooking and baking.
- Contains all 8 essential amino acids, making it a perfect source of protein.

Granola with banana and yoghurt

SERVES ❶

1 medium banana (80 g peeled weight)
100 ml low fat natural yoghurt
25 g granola

HOW TO PREPARE:

1 Peel and slice a banana in a bowl.

2 Pour yoghurt over the banana and mix well.

3 Sprinkle granola on top and serve.

NOTE: As granola is so high in calories, it is important to weigh it. Otherwise your calorie count could end up higher.

APPROXIMATELY ❷❻❿ KCAL PER SERVING

Lunch recipes

Low fat turkey and coleslaw wrap

SERVES **4**

300 g/2-3 carrots
500 g/$^1/_2$ Savoy cabbage
120 g/2-3 small red onions
300 ml low fat natural yoghurt
2 tbsp readymade horseradish sauce
100 ml apple juice
240 g turkey breast
low calorie spray oil
2 tbsp soy sauce
2 large tortilla wraps halved or 4 low calorie wraps

HOW TO PREPARE:

1   Wash and thinly peel the carrots and remove both ends.

2   Remove outer leaves of cabbage and wash the individual leaves.

3   If you have a household appliance to shred vegetables, shred the onion, carrots and cabbage. Otherwise you will need to shred them by hand using a knife and a grater.

4   Mix together natural yoghurt, horseradish sauce and apple juice in a bowl.

5   Add the yoghurt mixture to the vegetables and mix well.

6   Shred your turkey breast into thin slices.

7   Spray a non-stick pan with low calorie spray oil.

8   Cook your turkey for 5-10 minutes until cooked through.

9   Add some soy sauce to the turkey.

10   Serve your turkey in a wrap with your homemade coleslaw on the side.

NOTE: If making this dish for one, you could prepare the coleslaw on a Sunday and then use it during the week for your salads.

APPROXIMATELY **300** KCAL PER SERVING

Creamy salmon quiche

I used to make a lot of pies and quiches when I was a housewife with small children. In fact, I put on a few extra kilos as a result! I have changed this recipe so that the calories per portion are actually quite low. Be careful when you are eating out as a regular quiche is not low in calories!

SERVES 8

Base
4 tbsp Dr Eva's healthy spread (see recipe on p.207)
60 g oats (divided)
110 g wholemeal flour
pinch of salt

Filling
350 g/3 courgettes
300 g/1 large fennel
100 g/1 leek
3–4 tbsp low fat milk
100 g sliced smoked salmon
2 medium eggs
100 g low fat crème fraîche
100 g low fat feta cheese

tinfoil

HOW TO PREPARE:

1   Put Eva's spread in a bowl and add 40 g oats and wholemeal flour and pinch of salt. Knead together.

2   When it becomes a dough, add another 20 g oats to ensure the mixture is not too wet.

3   Place dough in a non-stick quiche dish (approximately 25 cm/10 inches in diameter).

4   Using your hands, evenly spread the dough on the base of the dish. Try to ensure that the thickness of the base is even so that it will hold all of the ingredients in the end. Mould the dough around the edge of the dish, approximately 5 cm/2 inches in height to form a crust.

5   Place dish in the fridge and begin to prepare your filling.

6   Wash courgettes. Cut in rounds.

7   Wash both the fennel and the leek and slice them in half. Slice both thinly.

8   Place these vegetables in a non-stick pan with the milk and cook on a medium heat until soft. Cook initially covered and then remove lid to allow excess water to evaporate.

9   Allow to cool.

10 Pre-heat the oven to 200 °C.

11 When vegetables are cool, remove the base from the fridge and fill with vegetables.

12 Chop salmon finely and add to filling.

OPTION: If you do not wish to use salmon, you could use 4 turkey rashers, chop finely and fry.

13 Crack 2 eggs and beat together with crème fraîche in a bowl. Pour over filling and smooth out evenly using a spatula.

14 Crumble feta cheese and sprinkle across the top of the quiche.

15 Place in preheated oven for 25 minutes uncovered.

16 After 25 minutes, cover the dish with tinfoil and place back in the oven for a further 15–20 minutes depending on your oven.

17 Serve with a green salad, e.g. lettuce, cucumber and celery, etc.

APPROXIMATELY ❷❺❺ KCAL PER SERVING

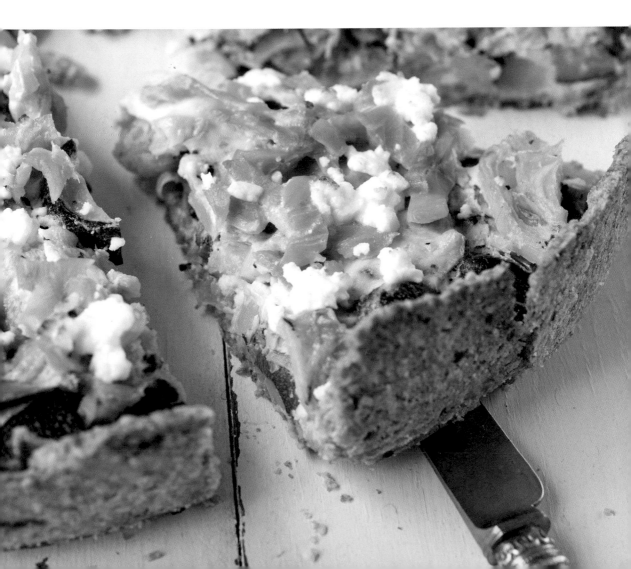

Niçoise salad

I often make this salad at home or if we are on holidays. It is so easy and filling and everyone likes it. If you have some left over, it is easy to keep for the next meal.

SERVES ❶

300 g fine French beans
1 egg
Iceberg lettuce
100 g/1 tomato, sliced
70 g/1 small tin of tuna in brine

Salad dressing
1 tbsp olive oil
1 tbsp balsamic vinegar
½ tsp mustard
black pepper to taste
pinch of salt

HOW TO PREPARE:

1   Steam French beans for 8–10 minutes in a steamer.

2   Boil and then slice the egg.

3   To prepare salad dressing, mix the ingredients together in a bowl.

4   Place French beans on a dish of lettuce. Slice the tomato and place over beans.

5   Add tuna and sliced egg. Drizzle with salad dressing.

APPROXIMATELY ❸❶❶ KCAL PER SERVING

Leek and potato soup with a vegetable you do not like

This is an ideal recipe to help get rid of food dislikes and introduce new flavours and choice into the diet.

SERVES **8**

800 g potatoes
400 g/2–3 big leeks
1 tbsp olive oil
700 ml boiling water from the kettle
1 vegetable stock cube or 15 ml Swiss vegetable vegan bouillon
a vegetable you do not like, for example 400 g courgettes, chopped
250 ml low fat milk
fresh ground black pepper (optional)

HOW TO PREPARE:

1 Peel and chop the potatoes into cubes. Slice the leeks.

2 Heat oil in a pot. Add leeks and simmer until soft.

3 Add potatoes and 700 ml of boiling water from the kettle.

4 Add one vegetable stock cube or 15 ml Swiss vegetable vegan bouillon.

5 Add your chosen vegetable, which you do not like (washed and chopped).

6 Simmer for 10–15 minutes. In the last few minutes add 250 ml low fat milk.

7 Liquidise if preferred.

8 Add black pepper (optional).

Examples of vegetables you can use: courgettes, cauliflower, broccoli, cabbage, green peppers, fennel and turnip.

Examples of vegetables not to use: carrots, parsnip and onion.

OPTION: Serve with 3 Finn Crisp crackers and 1 triangle of low fat soft cheese.

APPROXIMATELY **231** KCAL PER SERVING

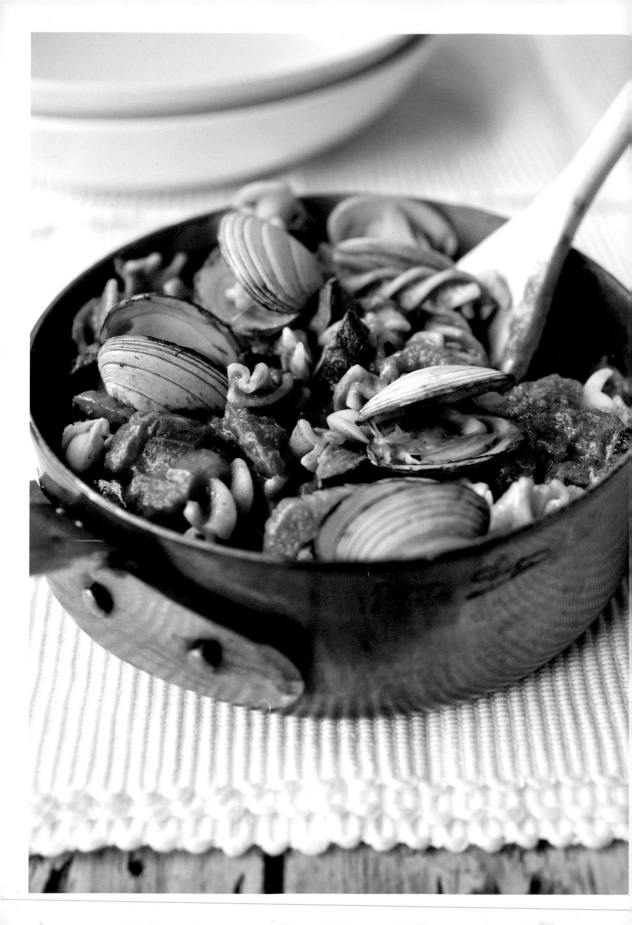

Cockle pasta

Italians love their seafood. Always keep some seafood in your freezer so you can come up with a dish in no time.

SERVES **4**

250 g/1 fennel
1 tbsp vegetable vegan Swiss bouillon/vegetable stock cube
100 ml water
300 g wholewheat fusilli pasta
150 g/1 courgette
400 g/1 (400 g) can of tomatoes
270 g cockles (frozen)
2–4 garlic cloves (depending on taste)
100 g low fat soft cheese

HOW TO PREPARE:

1 Wash your fennel and chop thinly.

2 Melt the vegetable Swiss bouillon or stock cube in 100 ml water.

3 Cook fennel in a non-stick pan in the stock for approximately 5 minutes (it takes longer to cook than the other vegetables).

4 Place your pasta in a pan and cook as per instructions.

5 Wash courgette and slice down the middle. Cut it in thin half moons and add to pan with fennel.

6 Add tin of tomatoes to the pan and cover. Allow to simmer for 5 minutes.

7 Wash your cockles and add to pan.

8 Peel and crush garlic. Add to pan.

9 When pasta is cooked, drain it and add to pan. Mix well.

10 Add the cheese to pan and mix well until melted and serve.

OPTION: You can substitute clams or mussels for the cockles.

APPROXIMATELY **310** KCAL PER SERVING

Dinner recipes

Puy lentil stew

A tasty vegetarian option. Cooking the baby onions whole gives the meal a new slant.

SERVES 4

240 g green lentils (Puy)
500 g baby onions
400 g/4 carrots
400 g/bunch of celery sticks
5 garlic cloves
4 bacon rashers (streaky or plain)
sprig of rosemary
1 tbsp olive oil
100 ml red wine

2 tbsp soy sauce
1 vegetable stock cube/15 ml Swiss
    vegetable vegan bouillon
500 ml boiling water from kettle
freshly ground black pepper
2 bay leaves
1 tbsp balsamic vinegar
2 tbsp chopped parsley

HOW TO PREPARE:

1 If time is available, soak lentils in water for 4–5 hours as this will speed up cooking. Lentils can also be used without soaking, just rinse under water.

2 Peel onions and leave whole. Peel and chop the carrots, celery and garlic. Remove visible fat from rashers and cut into thin strips.

3 Tie the rosemary together with a piece of thread. This will make it easier to remove before serving.

4 Heat oil in a saucepan, then add rashers. Then add onion and cook until brown. Cover for a few minutes.

5 Add the lentils, carrots, celery, wine, soy sauce, garlic, stock cube, 500 ml boiling water, pepper, rosemary, bay leaves and balsamic vinegar. Stir continuously.

6 Turn down heat and simmer for 20–30 minutes until lentils and onions are soft.

7 Remove the rosemary and bay leaf and stir in chopped parsley.

APPROXIMATELY 382 KCAL PER SERVING

Guinness casserole

Being a foreigner in Ireland, I had to do a dish with Guinness! I cooked this for my relatives when they came over for a visit. It's a great way of getting your 5 a day.

SERVES ❹

600 g rib steak
150 g/1 onion, peeled
400 g/4 carrots
300 g/2 peppers
150 g/1 courgette
400 g baby potatoes
1 tbsp olive oil
500 ml/1 pint of Guinness
1 beef stock cube
250—500 ml boiling water from the kettle
1 tsp whole black peppercorns
4 garlic cloves, peeled and crushed
2 bay leaves

HOW TO PREPARE:

1 Cut the steak into cubes. Wash the vegetables and chop the onions, carrots, peppers and courgettes into chunks. Wash baby potatoes. Do not peel them. Cut them in half.

2 Heat oil in a large non-stick pan or cast-iron ovenproof pot. Add the steak and onions and cook until brown.

3 Pour the Guinness into the pan. Add the beef stock cube and the water from the kettle (500 ml water needed if cooking on the stove and 250 ml is needed if cooking in oven).

4 Add carrots, peppers, courgettes, potatoes, black peppercorns, garlic and bay leaves. Stir. Do not cover but stir regularly. If you are cooking in the oven, then cover with lid and place in preheated oven.

5 Simmer for 40 minutes until vegetables are soft.

NOTE: This recipe can also be cooked in the oven at 200 °C for 1 hour + 15—40 depending on how the vegetables are cut. The dish must be covered with a lid.

APPROXIMATELY ❹❷❹ KCAL PER SERVING

Monkfish wrapped in bacon with stir-fried vegetables

Monkfish is not cheap but it is really delicious. Save it either for a special occasion or if you feel like treating yourself while 'on a diet'.

SERVES ❹

400 g/4 carrots
150 g/1 red pepper
150 g/1 yellow pepper
light spray oil
800 g fresh monkfish, cut in 4 portions
4 slices of Parma ham
1 tbsp olive oil
2 tbsp soy sauce
400 g French beans
2 tbsp oyster sauce
1 tbsp ginger, finely chopped

tinfoil

HOW TO PREPARE:

1 Preheat oven to 200 ˚C.

2 Chop the carrots and peppers into strips.

3 Line a baking tray with tinfoil. Spray with oil to prevent the fish sticking.

4 Wrap the monkfish in the Parma ham and place on the baking tray. Wrap the ends of the tinfoil and pinch to create a parcel to seal.

5 Place the monkfish in the oven to bake for 8–10 minutes.

6 While the fish is in the oven, stir-fry your vegetables. First, heat the oil in a wok and then add the vegetables starting with the carrots and French beans. Cook for a few minutes and then add the peppers. Cover and cook for 3 minutes.

7 Stir in the soy sauce, oyster sauce and grated ginger. Cover and cook for a further 3 minutes.

8 When the monkfish is cooked, remove from the oven, open the tinfoil parcel and serve with the stir-fried vegetables. If using rashers, make sure they are cooked thoroughly.

APPROXIMATELY ❸❶❻ KCAL PER SERVING

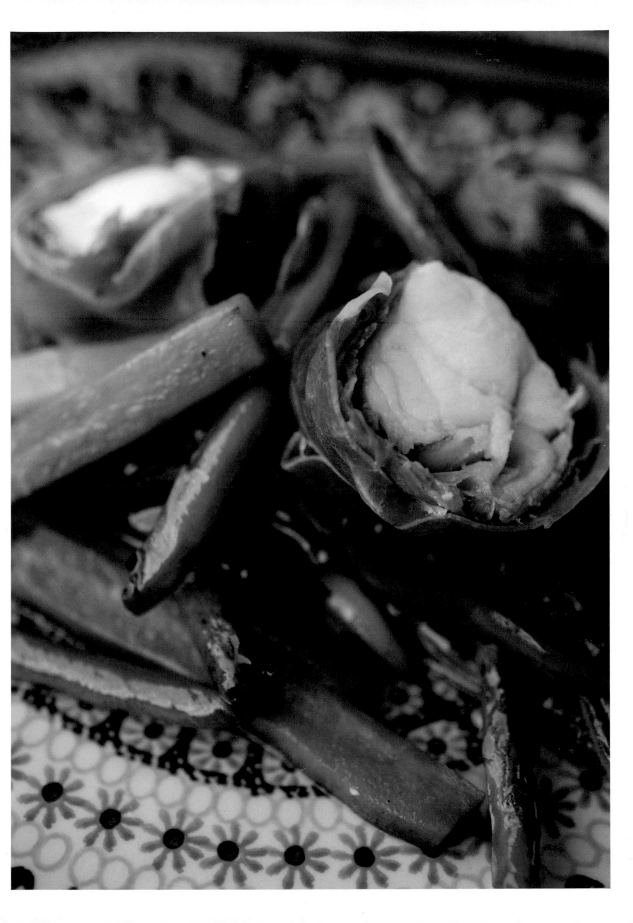

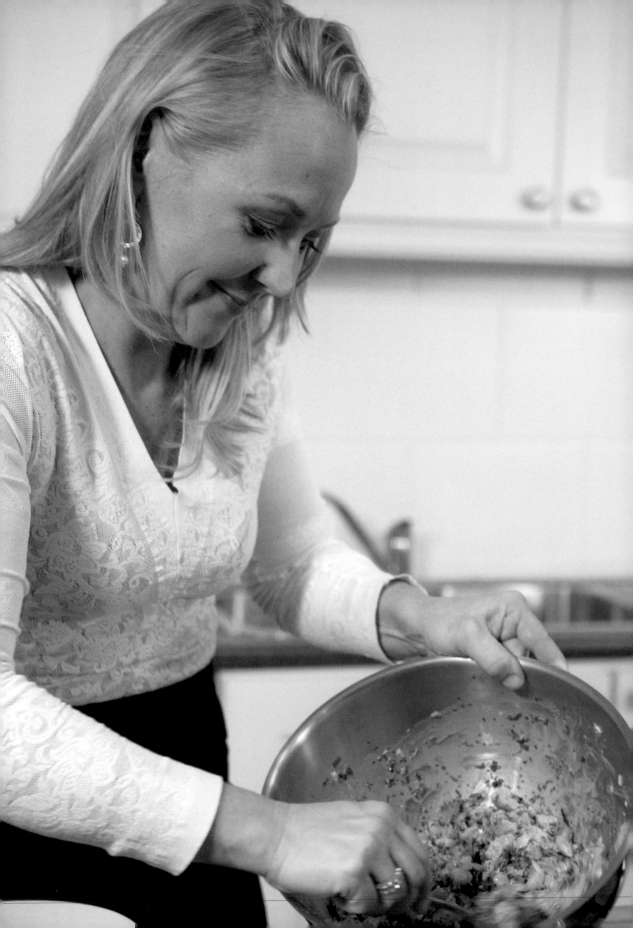

Indian chicken with herbs and couscous

I really love the green-coloured sauce and the smell is gorgeous—overall a truly appealing dish. You can cook the chicken in this way and serve it with steamed vegetables instead of couscous, if you prefer.

SERVES **4**

Marinade
400 g chicken fillets, cut into
   strips
1 lemon, squeezed
1 tsp salt
2 tsp grated ginger
2 tsp garlic paste
2 tsp vegetable oil
1 tsp crushed black pepper

Purée
50 g fresh mint leaves
150 g fresh coriander
100 g organic yoghurt
2 garlic cloves, crushed
2 green chillies, chopped
3 tsp olive oil
salt to taste

Couscous
200 g couscous
250 ml boiling water
2 tbsp Swiss vegetable vegan
   bouillon
2 punnets cherry tomatoes,
   cut in half
1 cucumber, chopped
4 pears, peeled and sliced
coriander to garnish

light spray oil
cling film

HOW TO PREPARE:

1 To prepare the marinade: Mix all ingredients in a bowl. Cover chicken with marinade and place in the fridge for 1 hour or prepare the night before.

2 To prepare the purée : Place all the ingredients in a food processor (or a hand blender can be used) and mix.

3 Mix half the purée with the marinated chicken.

4 Heat a large non-stick pan. Spray with the oil, add chicken and cook until chicken is done.

5 In the meantime place the couscous in a bowl. Cover with 250 ml boiling water mixed with the Swiss vegetable bouillon. Cover with cling film and set aside for 5–10 minutes until fluffy.

6 Separate grains with fork immediately. Add tomatoes, cucumber and pears.

7 Serve the chicken with the couscous mixture and drizzle the other half of the purée over the meal.

8 Garnish with coriander.

APPROXIMATELY **381** KCAL PER SERVING

Grilled tuna steak with Italian peperonata

My children thought tuna was chicken when they were small. This dish is a great way to introduce fish to anybody who thinks they hate seafood. Everybody's taste buds can be changed.

SERVES ❹

600 g/4 peppers
200 g/1 onion, peeled
6 garlic cloves, peeled
2 tbsp olive oil (divided)
400 g/1 (400g) can whole tomatoes
10 olives (optional)
2 tbsp soy sauce
1 tsp chopped chillies (optional)
1 tbsp tomato purée
1 tbsp tapenade (optional)
225 ml boiling water (divided)
100 g couscous
480 g fresh tuna, cut into 4 steaks

cling film

HOW TO PREPARE:

1 Wash the peppers. Cut them in strips and slice the onion.

2 Heat 1 tablespoon of oil in a large non-stick pan.

3 Add the onion and peppers and fry for a few minutes.

4 Add tomatoes, olives, soy sauce, chillies, tomato purée, tapenade and garlic.

5 Add 100 ml boiling water from kettle if needed.

6 Simmer for 10–15 minutes, covered with the lid initially.

7 Place couscous in an oven dish. Add 125 ml boiling water and cover with cling film. Leave for 5–10 minutes until most of the water has absorbed. Then separate grains with a fork.

8 Coat tuna steak in the remaining oil.

9 Heat grill pan over very high heat. Place the oiled tuna steaks on the pan and cook for 2–3 minutes on each side. This will yield a rare texture. For 'medium', cook for a further 2 minutes on each side.

10 Serve tuna with couscous and pepper mixture.

APPROXIMATELY ❸❺❺ KCAL PER SERVING

Madras lamb curry

I am not particularly fond of lamb myself but I know many people are. The lamb taste in this dish is slightly disguised by the curry flavour. This is perfect for any novice chef.

SERVES **4**

700 g celeriac
300 g French beans
400 g broccoli
150 g/1 large onion
1 tbsp olive oil
600 g lamb loin chop cut into thin
  strips removing visible fat

4 garlic cloves, crushed
1–2 tsp Madras curry powder according
  to taste
3 tbsp soy sauce
1 Swiss vegetable vegan bouillon stock
  cube
300 ml boiling water from kettle

HOW TO PREPARE:

1 Wash, peel and chop the vegetables.

2 Heat the oil in a large non-stick pan. Add the lamb, garlic, onion and the Madras curry powder. Stir.

3 Then add the soy sauce, celeriac, stock cube and boiling water.

4 Cover and simmer for 20–25 minutes, stirring occasionally.

5 Add the broccoli and French beans for the last 10 minutes.

APPROXIMATELY **481** KCAL PER SERVING

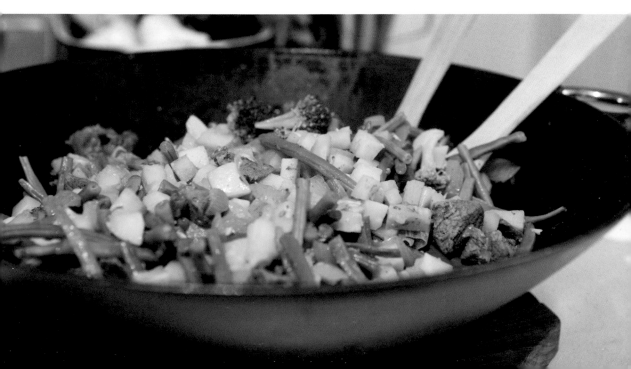

Thai green turkey curry

If you like curry, you will love this. Turkey keeps the fat content low and the calories down.

SERVES ❹

300 g/½ butternut squash or 300 g/3 carrots
300 g celeriac
150 g/1 onion
300 g/2 green peppers
25 g peppadews
600 g turkey
1 tbsp olive oil
1 Swiss vegetable vegan bouillon stock cube dissolved in 500 ml of boiling water
1 tbsp Thai green curry paste
2 kaffir lime leaves
2 tbsp soy sauce
3 garlic cloves, crushed
300 g French beans

HOW TO PREPARE:

1 Peel butternut squash, celeriac and onion and remove pips from the pepper. Cut all the vegetables in thin strips paying special attention to celeriac and butternut squash. You want them to cook as quickly as the onion and the pepper.

2 Finely chop the peppadews and cut turkey into strips.

3 Heat the oil in a wok. Add celeriac and butternut squash and cover for 2 minutes to keep moisture inside.

4 Add the onions and peppers, cover and cook for 1 minute.

5 Add vegetable stock, stir and add curry paste and lime leaves and cover again. You want the spices to activate under the heat and the flavours to soak into the vegetables. Cook for 3–4 minutes.

6 Add turkey, peppadews, soy sauce, crushed garlic and French beans.

8 Cover and simmer for 5–7 minutes until turkey is thoroughly cooked. Stir occasionally.

9 Remove the lime leaves before serving.

APPROXIMATELY ❸❼❶ KCAL PER SERVING

Beef au vin à la Eva

I am not a great connoisseur of French cuisine but this is my take on a classic French dish.

SERVES ❹

600 g sirloin steak
200 g/2 onions
300 g mushrooms
400 g/4 carrots
400 g broccoli
1 tbsp olive oil
1 tbsp crushed garlic
2 bay leaves

1 beef stock cube dissolved in 250 ml
   boiling water from the kettle
400 g/1 (400 g) can of whole peeled tomatoes
pinch of salt and pepper
sprig of fresh rosemary
200 ml red wine (roughly a small bottle)
1½ tbsp cranberry sauce

HOW TO PREPARE:

1 Cut steak into strips. Wash and peel the vegetables and chop them into chunks.

2 Heat oil in a large pan, add the steak, onions and garlic.

3 When steak is browned, add all the vegetables.

4 Add the rest of the ingredients. Bring to the boil.

5 Simmer for 20–30 minutes. Stir regularly. Remove the rosemary and bay leaves.

APPROXIMATELY ❹⓿⓿ KCAL PER SERVING

Chapter 9:
How the body metabolises energy

IN ORDER TO lose weight we need to cut down our daily food intake. In other words we have to create a negative energy balance. This must be done in a way that our body gets all the essential nutrients but does not get enough 'fuel', so it starts burning the existing fat reserves. You don't need to become a food science professional but basic knowledge is required so that in the future you will also know how to maintain your new healthy weight.

Food contains nutrients. Some nutrients contain energy (fuel); some do not but are still very important, for example fibre, water, mineral salts, trace elements and vitamins. These micronutrients are essential because the body needs them in different chemical reactions. Too small an intake of any of these can result in disease or poor functioning of the body. Foods that contain energy (expressed as kilocalories) are basically proteins, carbohydrates and fats (lipids). These are also called macronutrients and their main function is to provide energy but they are also needed for growth and repair.

When we eat something, it starts to break down into its basic constituents and is absorbed as follows:

- Proteins are absorbed as peptides and amino acids.
- Carbohydrates are broken down and are eventually absorbed as monosaccharides.
- Fats are absorbed as monoglycerides and fatty acids.

Protein

We need protein to produce new cells in our body to replace dead cells (e.g. skin and injured areas) and build our body (e.g. muscle, hair). Protein is essential for our wellbeing. Usually we get enough protein in our diet but the first signs of deficiency are that hair and nails stop growing as quickly, and wounds don't heal easily.

Low protein intake could be detrimental to your bone health. Dietary protein intakes at or below 0.8 g/kg of body weight have been associated with a reduction in intestinal calcium absorption. In the Developed World people are not usually deficient in protein when they are not trying to lose weight. But when people 'start a diet', their diet often becomes deficient in protein or they get far too much of it. When dietary protein is increased to 2 g/kg, it can induce hypercalciuria. This means your body loses calcium. So you have to make sure your diet includes a balanced amount of protein.

Proteins can be obtained from vegetable or animal sources. Proteins are made from long chains of amino acids. Some of these amino acids can be made by the body while others can only be obtained from food and are called 'essential amino acids'. Meat, fish, dairy and grains contain high quantities of amino acids but only eggs have a complete and balanced mixture of these amino acids.

The recommended daily intake of protein is 0.8 g/kg of body weight per day. An athlete could need up to 1.8 g/kg of body weight a day. People are not usually deficient in protein and in fact an average adult eats approximately 1–1.5 g/kg of body weight a day. A child's diet should contain at least 60 g of protein while an adolescent needs a minimum of 90 g. The minimum for a woman is 55 g per day while for a man it is 70 g per day.

We should get 15–30 per cent of our total daily calories from protein. As 1 g of protein contains 4 kcal, on an average maintenance diet we need about 300–600 kcal, or in practical terms 50–100 g of protein per day.

Generally speaking we can say that proteins are low glycaemic. However, it would depend a lot on the type of food that it is held in (and how it is prepared).

Remember, protein will only account for a moderate percentage of the food. Meat typically contains about 30 per cent protein. You will get 10 g of protein in 30 g of meat, 80 g of white fish, 50 g of chicken, 85 g of egg. For example, one 150 g chicken fillet will give you 30 g protein.

You can also get protein from broccoli, spinach, tofu, cottage cheese, chickpeas, lentils, beans and rice (listed in order of protein content—highest to lowest).

Carbohydrates

Carbohydrates are foods that break down into 'sugars' during digestion. They are the easiest and quickest form of energy for our bodies to use. In fact, most of the energy we need to move and think comes from carbohydrates. When we talk about 'sugar' in this context, we are not referring only to something sweet we add to our tea but to the final substance that ends up in the bloodstream after digestion—blood sugar. The richest sources of carbohydrates are bread, cereals, potatoes, rice, pasta, fruit, milk and of course sugar itself. Glucose is the purest form of carbohydrate and can be used as an energy source immediately while other carbohydrates have to be converted to a usable form in the liver. So, it is quite understandable that if glucose is eaten, sugars are rapidly released, creating a sudden and quick increase in blood sugar levels.

All carbohydrates are therefore not the same, because their absorption rate varies and this affects our bodies. There are those that enter the bloodstream very quickly and those that enter very slowly. When you eat sugar or sugary foods and drinks, like sweets or fizzy drinks, the sugar enters your blood very quickly, giving you a jolt of energy. Foods like wholemeal bread, apples and milk contain carbohydrates that are absorbed more slowly, which give a slow release of energy into the bloodstream.

So, what happens when we eat predominantly 'quick release carbohydrates'? Well, the quick burst of energy these carbohydrates give doesn't last very long and you soon feel hungry. You could spend all day trying to keep your energy up with sugary foods, eating more and more. Unfortunately, because you are not using up this energy, it then gets stored as fat and you start to notice that you are always tired and are gaining weight. What you really want is a slow and steady release of sugar into the blood so that your energy levels remain high for longer without having to eat as much. The amount of energy available to the body is also more controlled and you have a greater chance of using it before it gets stored as fat. We should therefore aim to eat fewer 'quick release' carbohydrates and more 'slow release' carbohydrates. The measure of how rapidly a carbohydrate food increases the blood sugar is called the Glycaemic Index, as explained in Chapter 3.

It is important to distinguish between the bad and good carbohydrates. I don't really like the terms 'bad' or 'good' as I believe in moderation in everything, but in this case I refer to 'bad' carbohydrates as being high glycaemic and good carbohydrates as being low glycaemic. This is not to be confused with the classical grouping of carbohydrates into 'simple' or 'complex', which was based on the chemical structure. We used to think that simple carbohydrates (like fructose) were quickly absorbed into the bloodstream and complex carbohydrates (like bread) were absorbed more slowly because of their more complex chemical structure. But this is not the case! To have a better understanding of this it helps to take a closer look at the chemical structure of carbohydrates. Technically speaking we divide them into monosaccharides, disaccharides and polysaccharides.

Monosaccharides (single sugar units):

Glucose, fructose and galactose

Disaccharides (two sugar units):

Sucrose or table sugar (glucose + fructose)

Lactose or milk sugar (glucose + galactose)

Maltose (glucose + glucose)

Polysaccharides (more than two sugar units):

Starch

Cellulose (fibre) non-starch polysaccharides

The monosaccharides and disaccharides are the 'simple' sugars and the polysaccharides are the 'complex' sugars. However, there is a significant difference in the rate of absorption (Glycaemic Index) between fructose and glucose as well as between starch and cellulose (fibre), etc. Using this as the basic rule for diet selection is therefore obviously flawed.

How much and which type of carbohydrates we should eat will continue to be contentious. The typical 'government issue' food pyramid and current nutritional guidelines recommends 6 or more servings a day from the base level. This would include predominantly carbohydrates that are easily absorbed like bread and potato (high glycaemic carbohydrates). This type of carbohydrate is also not particularly nice to eat in its basic form so all sorts of things are added to it and it's prepared in various ways to make it tastier, e.g. deep frying to make chips or spreading butter and jam on bread. We are not doing ourselves any favours by this. In contrast, the carbohydrates that are absorbed less rapidly (low glycaemic), such as carrots or broccoli, are quite palatable simply steamed or even raw or may require only a touch of something 'bad' to spice them up.

Then there is the standard recommendation to eat more fruit. Here again it is important to be able to choose the right 'slow energy release' fruit, like apples and oranges. You should limit fruit like grapes, bananas and dates, which contain glucose—a fast-release energy and high Glycaemic Index.

Our body needs energy, and carbohydrates are a good efficient source for immediate use. However, if the carbohydrates are not used, the excess energy gets stored as fat.

The nutritional value of hot drinks

Hot drinks vary significantly in nutritional value. This often depends on how they are made and whether there are any extra toppings, such as whipped cream. It is easy to forget that hot drinks contribute to our daily calorie intake. For example, consuming two whole milk lattes a day provides approximately 3,164 kcal per week! This is before we even account for the high fat, high calorie snacks, such as muffins and pastries, that often accompany the coffees.

The table opposite outlines the calorie, fat, carbohydrate, protein and caffeine content of various popular hot drinks.

As you can see, there is a significant difference between the calorie and fat content of many of the drinks depending on their ingredients. Hot drinks such as lattes, cappuccinos and hot chocolates, which are made with whole milk, are higher in calories and fat than those made with skimmed milk.

By choosing low fat versions of your preferred hot drink and avoiding extra toppings, you can reduce your calorie and fat intake considerably and still enjoy your favourite beverage.

With coffee being one of the most popular hot drinks consumed worldwide, it is interesting to note that recent research carried out in Sweden has actually found that habitual coffee consumption could potentially reduce the risk of stroke. In this particular study it was found that women who consumed more than one cup of coffee daily had a lower risk of stroke compared with women who consumed less than one cup of coffee daily. The risk of stroke appeared to be higher among women with low or no consumption of coffee.

Fats or lipids

We all know that butter is fat. We use butter to cook our foods and we spread it on our bread. Many years ago we had butter and olive oil but now we also have different types of margarines and oils that have been developed to 'lower your cholesterol' or be 'more heart friendly' and other wonderful claims.

Our body *needs* fat for cell membrane construction and for building hormones. We also need it for blood clotting. Our brain is 60 per cent fat! The majority of

	Calories (kcal)	Fat (g)	Carbohydrates (g)	Protein (g)	Caffeine (mg)
Tea (250 ml) with 30 ml whole milk	20	1	1.5	1	45
Tea (250 ml) with 30 ml semi-skimmed milk	14	0.5	1.5	1	45
Tea (250 ml) with 30 ml skimmed milk	10	0	1.5	1	45
Instant coffee (250 ml) with 30 ml whole milk	20	1	1.5	1	27–173
Instant coffee (250 ml) with 30 ml semi-skimmed milk	14	0.5	1.5	1	27–173
Instant coffee (250 ml) with 30 ml skimmed milk	10	0	1.5	1	27–173
Espresso (30 ml)	1	0	0	0	30–90
Americano (340 ml) with semi-skimmed milk (30 ml)	14	0.5	1.5	1	60–180
Latte (30 ml espresso with 340 ml whole milk)	226	11.3	17	11.3	30–90
Skinny latte (30 ml espresso with 340 ml semi-skimmed milk)	158	5.6	17	11.3	30–90
Latte (30 ml espresso with 340 ml skimmed milk)	119	0.17	17	11.3	30–90
Cappuccino (30 ml espresso and 340 ml whole milk)	226	11.3	17	11.3	30–90
Skinny cappuccino (espresso and 340 ml skimmed milk)	119	0.17	17	11.3	30–90
Hot chocolate (30 g chocolate with 340 ml whole milk and 30 ml whipped cream)	377	16	40	14	0
Hot chocolate (30 g chocolate with 340 ml skimmed milk)	230	2	39	13	0
Cadbury's Instant Hot Chocolate made with water (30 g)	111	1.77	22	1.89	0
Caffé mocha (30 g Cadbury's chocolate, espresso, 250 ml whole milk and 30 ml whipped cream)	319	13.5	35.7	11	30–90
Skinny Caffé Mocha (30 g Cadbury's chocolate, espresso, 250 ml skimmed milk)	200	1.77	34.5	10	30–90

our body's fat is in reserve as a 'store of energy' that can be used in a moment of energy scarcity.

Even though fats are necessary, our fat intake should be less than 30 per cent of our daily calorie requirements. The Japanese, who have the highest life expectancy in the world, with almost no excess weight or obesity, have only 15 per cent fat in their diet. The type of fat they eat is also relevant—the Japanese eat a lot of raw oily fish (sushi) that contains Omega 3 fatty acids.

SATURATED FATS

Saturated fats tend to be solid at room temperature and can be found naturally in many foods like butter, cheese, beef, lamb, chicken, ice cream, chocolate bars and milk. The more saturated fatty acids in the fat, the more heat is needed to make it liquid. For example, in the fridge butter is hard, margarine is soft and olive oil is liquid. Butter is high in saturated fats whereas olive oil has none. *Trans* fats are mostly created in food processing and manufacturing. This process (hydrogenation) is used to make the fats harder and is also used to increase the shelf life of foods like cakes, biscuits and crackers. These processed trans fats are unhealthy fats and should be avoided.

Both saturated and trans fats raise total cholesterol and LDL-cholesterol, which, in turn, raises your risk of heart disease. Trans fats are worse than saturated fats because not only do they raise the bad cholesterol, they also lower HDL (good) cholesterol. The list of foods that contain saturated and trans fats is long, making it difficult to avoid them completely. One way to cut back is to choose wisely when it comes to oils and fats that you add to foods in cooking or at the table. Use natural substances and avoid processed and unnatural margarines and spreads.

UNSATURATED FATS

Unsaturated fats have one or more double bonds holding them together. This type of fat is further classified into monounsaturated fatty acids (MUFAs) and polyunsaturated fatty acids (PUFAs) (mono having one double bond, poly having at least two double bonds).

Omega 3 and Omega 6 fatty acids are both polyunsaturated fats obtained from plants. These 'special' fats have been shown to protect the cardiovascular system against disease and be beneficial for the osteoarticular system (joints). However, many experts believe that the modern Western diet is weighted too much in favour of the Omega 6 series. Typical products providing Omega 6 fatty acids would be sunflower oil and their respective margarines. The suggestion is that we should in fact take more of the Omega 3 series. These are found in certain foods like oily fish (salmon, sardines, fresh tuna and mackerel), nuts and seeds, rapeseed oil and olive oil—these contain a lot of monounsaturated fats.

A good general guideline is that out of our total fat intake we should get at least 20 per cent of fats from mono and polyunsaturated fats, which provide the 3 and

6 Omega fatty acids. No more than one-third should be saturated. Some foods contain a lot of hidden fats. To reduce intake of saturated and trans fats, cut down on crackers, biscuits, crisps, chips, cakes, sweets and other packaged foods, eliminate lard and switch to low fat versions of milk, yoghurt and cheese. Rapeseed is the best oil for cooking, and sunflower and olive oils are also good choices—all are low in saturated fats and have a decent mix of MUFAs and PUFAs. As fish is lower in saturated fat than beef, pork and chicken, it is worth including it in your diet. Choose fish 2–3 times per week, one of which should be an oily fish, and limit your beef and pork to 1–2 servings per week.

COOKING AND FAT

How healthy your meals are depends on the type of cooking method you choose. Frying even healthy food can turn it into a cholesterol-raising fattening food. The best cooking methods to ensure that your food stays healthy are baking, grilling, microwaving, roasting and steaming (as long as you add little or no oil or fat!). Trim off any excess fat on meats and discard the skin on chicken before cooking as fat can seep into meat during cooking.

Fibre

There is an advertisement that goes something like this: 'Looking for an easier way to get enough fibre?' It continues '...just trying to get enough fibre can sometimes be a challenge on its own. After all, an adult needs at least 18 g of dietary fibre a day to keep their bowel healthy. In food terms, that's 13 portions of brown rice every day! Hardly a mouth-watering proposition, is it?' The advert then promotes an 'over the counter' medicine to relieve symptoms of constipation.

Why do we need a medicine when all we really need is to consume some fibre-rich vegetables? Current guidelines recommend that we should get 15 g of fibre per 1,000 kcal. So, for a normal diet of 2,000–2,500 kcal, the recommended daily quantity for fibre is at least 30 g! Most people don't even get the minimum 18 g of fibre a day.

When you are trying to lose weight and consuming about 1,200 kcal a day, it can be more difficult to fit 25–30 g of fibre into the diet. However, increased fibre intake can be advantageous, providing a larger serving but still with low calories.

Dietary fibre is made up of non-starch polysaccharides, which have such a complex structure that our digestive enzymes are unable to break them into smaller digestible particles and that's why they don't get absorbed and cannot be used as energy. Fruit (apples and oranges) and vegetables (broccoli, asparagus) that contain a high percentage of fibre will also help to slow down the release of sugar into the blood.

Fibre has no so-called 'nutritional value' because it cannot be absorbed but it is of crucial importance. Fibre gives you:

- **A sense of fullness—it bulks up meals without bulking up calories.**
- **Longer-lasting satiety—you feel fuller for longer.**
- **A lower glycaemic effect—it slows down the speed at which sugars are absorbed into the bloodstream, hence lowering the Glycaemic Index of food.**
- **Improved 'internal transit'—it keeps the bowels moving (studies have shown that a diet with adequate fibre can protect us from diseases like heart disease and colon cancer).**

To increase your daily fibre intake, choose wholemeal versions of starchy carbohydrates like pasta, crackers and bread. Choose a minimum of 5 servings of fruit and vegetables daily. Try eating your potatoes with their skins to get more fibre. Reading food labels can help you make better choices between types of breads, snacks and other foods.

People often choose 'salads' when they try to lose weight because of their low calorie content. They would typically be a combination of lettuce, tomatoes, cucumber and celery. These low calorie vegetables are very 'light' and even if you made a substantial quantity of this type of salad, the actual fibre content would still be very low. It is important to choose vegetables that have a high fibre content. Top of the list of the 'regular' vegetables are carrots and broccoli, but there are others that have much higher fibre content. To help you choose, I have compiled a table that gives you the 'fibre ratio' of foods.

Fibre ratio is a tool to compare the calorie efficiency of each gram of fibre. In other words, what is the best way to get fibre with the fewest calories. We must, however, also keep in mind that all the vegetables also contain protein (in varying proportions) especially beans, lentils, pulses, and the calories from these are predominantly from proteins.

These high protein vegetables (beans, lentils, pulses) could be used to provide the necessary protein as well as being an excellent source of fibre. The table opposite outlines the fibre ratio of some vegetables.

From this table, you can clearly see that the advertisement discussed previously used the worst fibre content example (brown rice) to promote its product!

	Fibre ratio g fibre/kcal	Fibre g/100 g	Calories kcal/100 g	Carbohydrates g/100 g
Fennel	0.21	2.3	11	1.5
Celery	0.15	1.2	8	0.8
Aubergines (raw)	0.13	2	15	2.2
Green cabbage	0.11	1.8	16	2.2
French beans	0.11	2.4	22	2.9
Runner beans	0.11	1.9	18	2.3
Carrots	0.1	2.5	24	4.9
Green peppers	0.1	1.8	18	2.6
Mushrooms	0.1	1.1	11	0.4
Broccoli	0.1	2.3	24	1.1
Brussels sprouts	0.09	3.1	35	3.5
Leeks	0.08	1.7	21	2.6
Parsnip	0.07	4.7	66	12.9
Lettuce (raw)	0.06	0.9	14	1.7
Courgette	0.06	1.2	19	2
Kidney beans	0.06	6.2	100	17.8
Cucumber (raw)	0.06	0.6	10	1.5
Cauliflower	0.06	1.6	28	2.1
Peas	0.06	4.5	79	10
Asparagus	0.05	1.4	26	1.4
Bean sprouts	0.05	1.3	25	2.8
Butter beans	0.05	5.2	103	18.4
Red peppers	0.05	1.7	34	7
Soya beans	0.04	6.1	141	5.1
Onions	0.04	0.7	17	3.7
Chickpeas	0.04	4.3	121	18.2
Mange-tout peas	0.03	0.8	26	3.3
Black eye beans	0.03	3.5	116	19.9
Potato (not new)	0.02	1.2	72	17
Lentils	0.01	3.8	297	16.9
Brown rice (raw)	0.01	1.9	357	81.3

Chapter 10:
Phase 3—
1,600 kcal diet

THIS PHASE IS similar to Phase 2 in that it is also based on healthy eating guidelines. On this phase the carbohydrate and dairy allowances are increased but this also increases the total calorie intake. Some people will find the increase in portion size more gratifying than previous phases.

As there is more food choice, meal options are more varied and interesting. When eating out, ordering is far easier at this stage because it is more flexible. However, this means it is easier to consume more calories than you should—which could effectively bring you up to the maintenance stage, so be careful. If your calorie intake continues to increase, you will find it very hard to lose weight.

Behaviour modification is a key component of this phase. Portion sizes need to be monitored, as do the addition of various sauces and dressings, to keep calorie intake under control. Snack options must still be healthy and low calorie but there is more choice on offer.

This phase is ideal for anyone who has a BMI in the overweight category (25–29). This is a balanced healthy eating plan that is very close to a maintenance plan but still maintains a small energy deficit. Very petite people may find it hard to lose weight on this plan and it may be more suitable as a maintenance plan for them. Women can expect to lose between 0.6–1 kg (1–2.2 lb) a week depending on size and activity levels, and similarly men can expect to lose up to 1.6 kg (4 lb) a week.

This diet can also be followed by anyone who has progressed through Phases 1 or 2 and now wishes to reintroduce more food choices into their diet to gradually move towards a maintenance plan. Alternatively you may choose this plan if you want to lose weight more slowly and gradually than on the 1,200 kcal phase. This phase is ideal for anyone who does strenuous exercise and can therefore have a higher calorie intake while still losing weight. It is also suitable as an initial phase for men who do not have much weight to lose and want to exercise.

Exercise

Regular exercise is essential to increase the energy deficit and speed up weight loss. Walking for 30 minutes will burn up a maximum of 250 calories. You should aim to walk further or start running so that you slowly increase your level of exertion, and don't stagnate.

Eating out

Eating out is far more manageable on this phase because you have a bigger calorie allowance to work with—but this is where the hidden danger lies, as you can easily forget you are on a diet. You can eat almost any type of food on this plan, but be particularly careful with portion size. Most restaurants serve double what we should really be eating. Remember, alcohol stimulates the appetite so is probably best avoided. To make things simpler, choose between a starter or a dessert or, if you wish to have all three courses, choose a salad as a starter and select a vinaigrette dressing. Be careful with dessert because you could be unknowingly eating your whole day's calorie allowance. Use the common sense and knowledge that you have obtained by this stage. Fruit salads and sorbets are the best dessert options. Try to avoid cream at all costs.

Meal options

Breakfast 300 kcal, Lunch 400 kcal, Dinner 600 kcal, Snacks 300 kcal

Breakfast
1. Karelian pastries
2. Apple crumble à la Eva
3. Fresh cherry tomato bruschetta
4. Egg à la coque

Lunch
You could alternatively have a filler soup with some (3–5) cracker breads and light soft cheese, or make a salad, depending on the calories. See the Soup section on p.191 and the Salad section on p.201.
1. Quick lunchtime pizza
2. Chickpea burgers with cucumber raita and green salad
3. Butternut squash and red lentil stew
4. Risotto with beetroot and fennel
5. Baked potato filled with Coronation salmon

Dinner
1. Pasta box with rainbow vegetables
2. Chilli con carne
3. Chicken goujons with sweet potato chips and tomato salad
4. Pasta carbonara à la Eva
5. Peppers stuffed with feta cheese and pine nuts
6. Four Seasons pizza à la Eva
7. Caprese omelette
8. Twice-baked potatoes

Snacks
You can choose 2 snacks (amounting to 300 kcal in total) each day. Ideally have 1 snack mid-morning and the other mid-afternoon. Some ideas are:
1. 1 tbsp walnuts mixed with 1 tbsp cashew nuts (189 kcal)
2. Strawberries with chocolate sauce: 150 g strawberries, 2 squares Bourneville melted—dip strawberries into chocolate (110 kcal)
3. Half a banana with 17 raspberries covered in low calorie yoghurt (125 kcal)
4. 30 g tortilla chips and 30 g guacamole (176 kcal)
5. 150 g low calorie natural or fruit yoghurt with 2 tbsp no added sugar muesli (169 kcal)
6. 1 slice of wholemeal bread toasted with 1 tbsp honey (129 kcal)

Filler soups (see section p.191)
1. Celeriac and apple soup
2. Fennel and orange soup
3. Hot mushroom soup
4. Red cauliflower soup
5. Hot fennel cauliflower soup
6. Mixed vegetable soup
7. Spicy cauliflower soup
8. Mild cinnamon cauliflower soup
9. Spinach soup
10. Broccoli soup
11. Green curry turnip soup

Nutrition and health facts

1 The most dangerous place to carry weight is around your middle: a woman's waist should be less than 80 cm (32 inches), and a man's less than 94 cm (37 inches) across the navel. A waistline of over 102 cm for a man and 88 cm for a woman carries a substantial risk to health.

2 Excess weight spreads: if your friends and family are overweight, then you are more likely to become overweight.

3 52 per cent of women on the island of Ireland are overweight.

4 Three times as many men and twice as many women are clinically obese compared with 1990 figures.

5 Today's 14-year-olds are about 19 kg (3 st) heavier than their grandmothers at the same age.

Top row, left to right: fresh cherry tomato bruschetta, Karelian pastries, quick lunchtime pizza; bottom row, left to right: butternut squash and red lentil stew, twice-baked potatoes, pasta box with rainbow vegetables

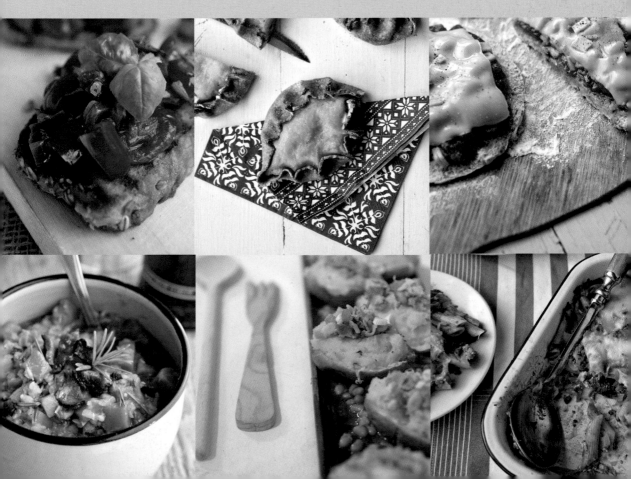

Breakfast recipes

Karelian pastries

Everybody eats Karjalan piirakka *in Finland. The original recipe is made with rice but the turnip filling makes them healthier!*

SERVES ❹ (MAKES 16 PASTRIES)

Pastry
200 g rye flour
50 g white flour
1 tsp salt
100 ml water

Filling
1 kg/1 turnip
salt

Egg spread
3 eggs
100 ml low fat sour cream
1 shallot

cling film

HOW TO PREPARE:

1 To make the pastry: Add the flour and salt to the water and mix into a solid, compact dough. Add more flour if it is not sticking. Roll dough out in a cylinder/sausage shape and cover in cling film. Place in fridge.

2 To make the filling: Peel a large turnip and chop into small pieces. Place in a pot and cover in water. Simmer for at least 40–50 minutes depending on how thick you cut it. Season with salt.

3 Take the dough from the fridge and divide it into 17 parts.

4 Roll into balls and flatten into cakes.

5 Sprinkle table and hands with rye flour. Roll the cakes into thin sheets with a rolling pin.

6 Drain excess water from turnip and mash with a potato masher.

7 Spread some turnip filling on each sheet and turn the edges partly over the filling and press to close.

8 Put on a baking tray and bake at 200 ˚C for 12 minutes.

9 Place the pastries, separated with greaseproof paper, in a bowl and cover with a towel to soften the crusts.

10 Now crack 3 eggs in a bowl and whisk together with sour cream.

11 Chop 1 shallot finely and add to egg mixture. Mix well.

12 Serve karelian pastries with egg spread, 4 pastries and 60 ml spread to a serving.

APPROXIMATELY ❷❼❽ KCAL PER SERVING (4 PASTRIES)

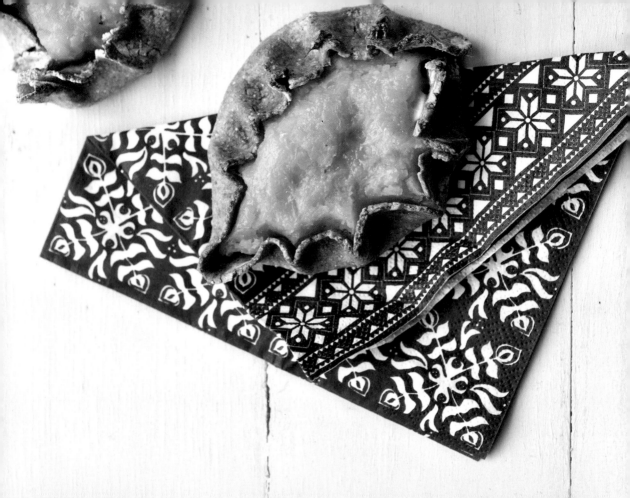

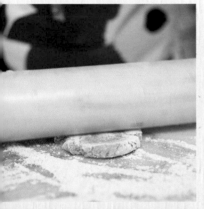

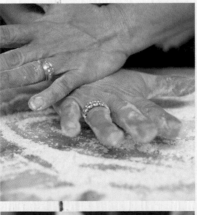

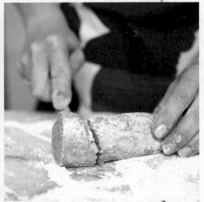

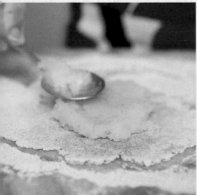

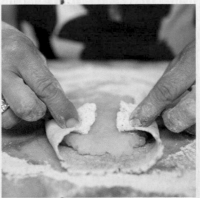

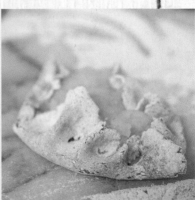

Apple crumble à la Eva

This recipe dates back to when I was eight! My mother always used to make this in autumn. I would make it at home in a big oven dish. If you want to overindulge, serve it with custard!

SERVES **1**

1 apple
oil to spray
40 g oats
low calorie sweetener
1 pot low fat low calorie vanilla yogurt

HOW TO PREPARE:

1 Preheat oven to 200 ˚C.

2 Peel the apple and remove the core. Slice the apple thinly.

3 Spray a small ovenproof dish with oil.

4 Place a layer of apples on the bottom of the dish and put a layer of oats over it.

5 Sprinkle with artificial sweetener and place the remaining apple slices over that. Finish off with a layer of oats and artificial sweetener.

6 Place in the preheated oven for 12–15 minutes.

7 Serve hot with vanilla yoghurt.

APPROXIMATELY **280** KCAL PER SERVING

Fresh cherry tomato bruschetta

A typical Italian starter that also makes an excellent breakfast!

light spray oil
50–60 g red onion
250 g cherry tomatoes
1 tbsp soy sauce
2 slices of wholegrain bread
1 tsp olive oil
2–4 garlic cloves, crushed (depending on your taste)
1 tbsp fresh basil
sprinkle of black pepper (optional)

HOW TO PREPARE:

1. Spray a non-stick pan with light spray oil.
2. Peel and chop your onion into small pieces and add to pan.
3. Wash your cherry tomatoes and, using a sharp knife, cut in quarters and add to pan. Cover to keep in the moisture and allow to sauté. Stir occasionally.
4. After 5 minutes add soy sauce. Allow to cook for a further 2 minutes.
5. Place your bread in toaster.
6. Mix your olive oil and crushed garlic in a bowl.
7. When the bread is toasted, layer with the oil and garlic mixture.
8. Top your toast with the tomato and onion mixture.
9. Place your fresh basil in a bowl and chop with a kitchen scissors. Sprinkle over your tomato mixture and serve.
10. You can add a pinch of black pepper to your bruschetta if you wish.

NOTE: some people do not like the tomato peel. However, it is a great source of fibre and has no calories so it is worth including.

APPROXIMATELY ❸❶❶ KCAL PER SERVING

Egg à la coque

A good old classic!

SERVES **1**

1 egg
2 slices of high fibre wholwheat bread (approx. 100 kcal) or 5 Finn Crisp
10 g Dr Eva's healthy spread (see p.207)

HOW TO PREPARE:

1 Boil egg for 3–4 minutes to keep it runny.

2 Toast your bread.

3 Remove the egg from saucepan and place in an eggcup—3 minutes should be sufficient to harden the egg white while leaving the egg yolk runny but warm.

4 Butter your bread with the healthy spread and cut into slices if you wish.

5 Remove the top of the egg and serve with the bread. A delicious way to eat this is to dip your toast into the egg yolk.

APPROXIMATELY **300** KCAL PER SERVING

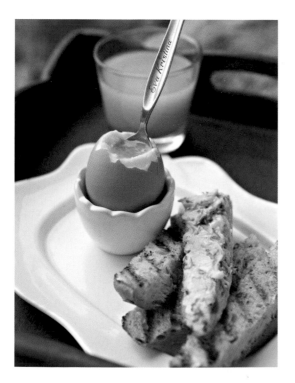

Lunch recipes

Quick lunchtime pizza

A homemade version is healthier than a takeaway.

1 wholegrain low calorie pitta bread
2 tbsp pasatta or tomato relish
2 slices of ham
2 slices of light cheese (single wrapped slices for convenience)
Bowl of filler soup (see Soup section on p.191)

HOW TO PREPARE:

1 Preheat grill.

2 Cut a wholegrain pitta in half to obtain 2 round bases and place on grill tray.

3 Cover both pitta halves with pasatta or relish.

4 Put a slice of ham on each pitta half.

5 Place a cheese slice on ham.

6 Place under the grill and allow cheese to melt.

7 Serve with a bowl of filler soup of your choice.

APPROXIMATELY ❸❺❾ KCAL PER SERVING

Chickpea burgers with cucumber raita and green salad

This is a really delicious vegetarian recipe.

SERVES 2

10 ml olive oil (divided)
200 g/2 carrots, grated
150g/1 onion, finely chopped
½ tsp chopped chillies in water
2 garlic cloves, crushed
¼ vegetable stock cube
a little boiling water from the kettle
1 can chickpeas (270 g drained weight),
   rinsed and drained
1 rye crackerbread
100 ml low fat natural yoghurt

1 egg
black pepper

Raita
¼ cucumber, chopped
¼ pepper, chopped
1 clove garlic, crushed
3–4 fresh mint leaves, finely chopped
100 ml natural yoghurt
pinch of paprika
baby gem leaves, to garnish

cling film

HOW TO PREPARE:

1 Heat the oil in a wok or non-stick pan. Add the grated carrot, chopped onion, chopped chillies, crushed garlic, vegetable stock cube and a little boiling water to the wok. Stir to combine, cover with a lid and cook on a medium heat for 5–10 minutes until the ingredients have softened.

2 While this is cooking, mash the chickpeas with a potato masher or an electric multi mixer.

3 Mix the mashed chickpeas with the cooked carrot and onion mixture in a bowl. Set aside to cool.

4 Under cling film, bash the rye crackerbread until it looks like breadcrumbs.

5 Beat the yoghurt and egg together with a fork in a bowl and stir in the bashed crackerbread. Set aside.

6 Once the chickpea, carrot and onion mix has cooled, stir in the yoghurt and crackerbread mixture. Add a pinch of black pepper.

7 Form little mini burgers from the mixture (4–6).

8 Heat 1 tablespoon of oil in your wok or non-stick pan on a medium heat and place your burgers on it to cook. Cover the pan and leave until fully cooked and browned. (Halfway during cooking turn the burgers so that they cook evenly on both sides.)

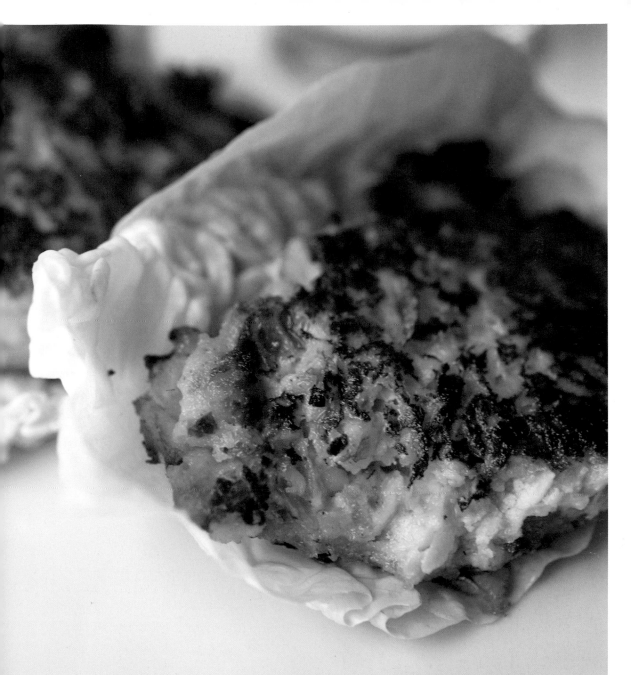

9   While they are cooking, make your raita by combining the cucumber, pepper, garlic, mint, yoghurt and pinch of paprika in a bowl.

10 To serve, place the cooked chickpea burgers on your baby gem leaves and spoon over the raita or serve the raita with it.

APPROXIMATELY ③⑨⓪ KCAL PER SERVING

Butternut squash and red lentil stew

My sister-in-law Gwynne taught me how to make this dish while we were living in South Africa. It's important to know how to cut butternut squash properly as it makes the preparation much easier. The original recipe has more bacon and cream in it but it is as nice without them!

SERVES ❹

100 g red lentils (uncooked)
1 tbsp olive oil
100 g bacon rashers, chopped thinly
150 g/1 onion, chopped
3 garlic cloves (optional)
600 g/½ large butternut squash, cut in cubes
½ vegetable stock cube dissolved in of 1 litre boiling water
2 tbsp soy sauce
1 sprig rosemary
black pepper

HOW TO PREPARE:

1 Soak the lentils in water for 30 minutes before you start cooking. Rinse.

2 Heat oil in a wok.

3 Add the chopped rashers, onion and garlic followed by the chopped butternut and lentils.

4 Pour in the vegetable stock mixture.

5 Introduce soy sauce and rosemary (wrapped in string) for extra flavour.

6 Bring stew to boil.

7 Turn down the heat to simmer for 25–35 minutes uncovered to obtain stew-like consistency.

8 When the butternut and lentils are soft, it's ready to eat.

9 Serve with 2 slices of Finn Crisp and Dr Eva's healthy spread (see p.207).

NOTE: You could drop the rashers to make the dish vegetarian.

APPROXIMATELY ❹❶❶ KCAL PER SERVING

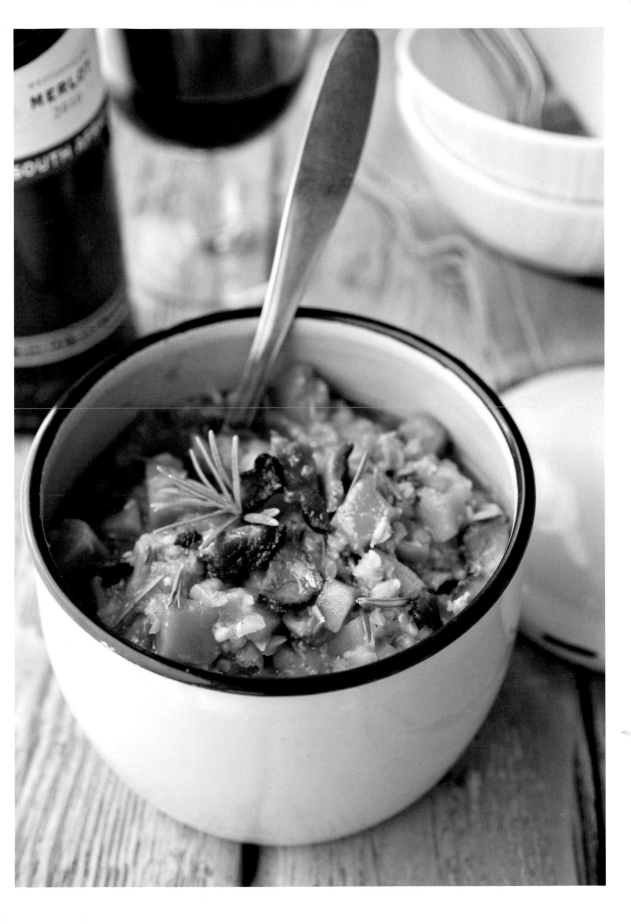

Risotto with beetroot and fennel

This dish is a combination of my student years in Italy and my Finnish love for beetroot.

SERVES **4**

1 tbsp olive oil
120 g/1 small onion
170 g small fennel/½ a large fennel
200 g/1 medium sized courgette
1 tbsp Swiss vegetable vegan bouillon/1 stock cube
1 litre boiling water from kettle
200 g Arborio risotto rice
2 tbsp soy sauce
300 g cooked beetroot
200 g tub of low fat crème fraîche
40 g parmesan cheese, grated

HOW TO PREPARE:

1   Heat the oil in a good non-stick pan.

2   Chop the onion and fennel finely and add to pan.

3   Wash the courgette. Chop both ends off and grate it thinly. Add to pan.

4   Fry until golden brown and partly cooked. If you need to, you can add a small amount of water to the pan. Cover and leave to simmer.

5   Boil the kettle and dissolve the vegetable bouillon/stock cube in a jug.

6   When the vegetables are partly cooked, add the risotto rice and soy sauce to the pan.

7   Slowly add small amounts of stock to the pan and stir continuously until the rice absorbs all the water. Then add some more of the stock and again stir until the rice has absorbed it. Repeat this process until all the stock has been used.

8   Cover the pan and allow to simmer for 15–20 minutes.

9   At this stage you can grate the beetroot and add it to the pan to heat it up.

10   When the risotto is almost ready, you can add the crème fraîche to the pan and stir well.

11   Serve the risotto on a serving dish and top with grated parmesan cheese.

APPROXIMATELY **400** KCAL PER SERVING

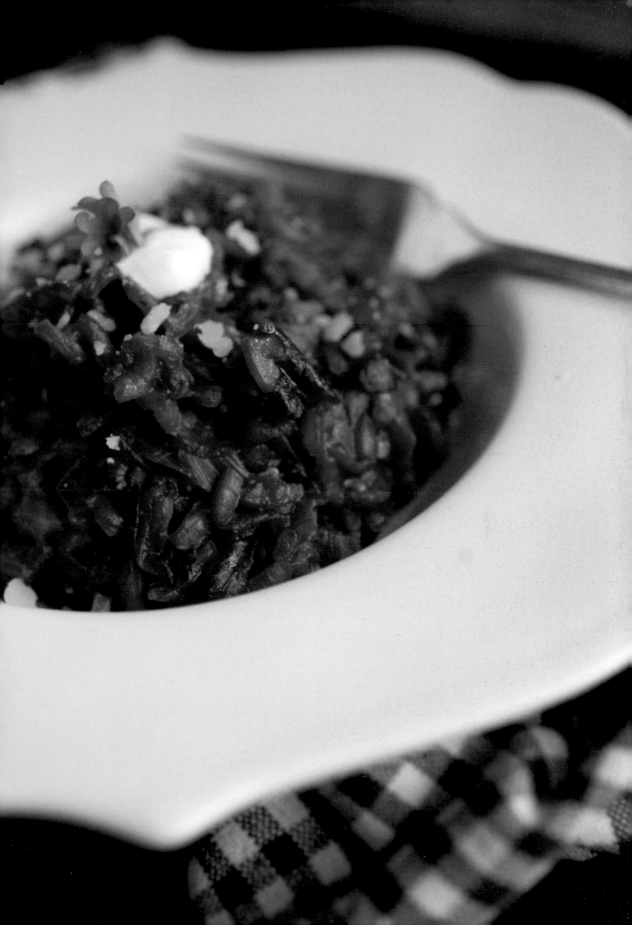

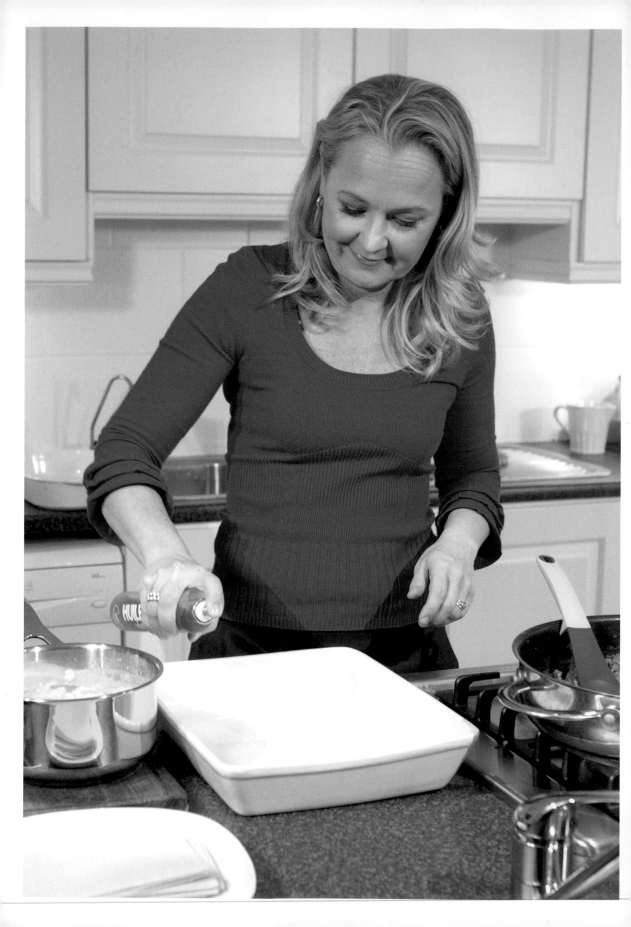

Baked potato filled with Coronation salmon

Most of the fibre in potatoes is in the skin. Wash the potatoes well so you end up eating the whole thing.

SERVES **1**

200–250 g/1 average baked potato
Filling
50 g smoked salmon (or alternatively you can use tuna)
20 g/1 shallot
50 g sweetcorn
50 ml natural yoghurt
50 g ricotta cheese
1 tsp curry powder
Side salad
150 g/1 baby gem or alternative lettuce

HOW TO PREPARE:

1 Preheat oven to 200 ˚C.

2 Scrub potato and pierce all over with a knife. Place in oven and bake until a knife penetrates easily, approximately 35 minutes.

3 While the potato is baking, prepare the filling.

4 Chop salmon and shallot in small pieces and place in a bowl.

5 Add the sweetcorn, natural yoghurt, ricotta cheese and curry powder and mix together using a fork.

6 Next wash and shred the lettuce.

7 When potato is ready, cut it partially in half and stuff with Coronation salmon mixture.

8 Serve with side salad.

APPROXIMATELY **400** KCAL PER SERVING

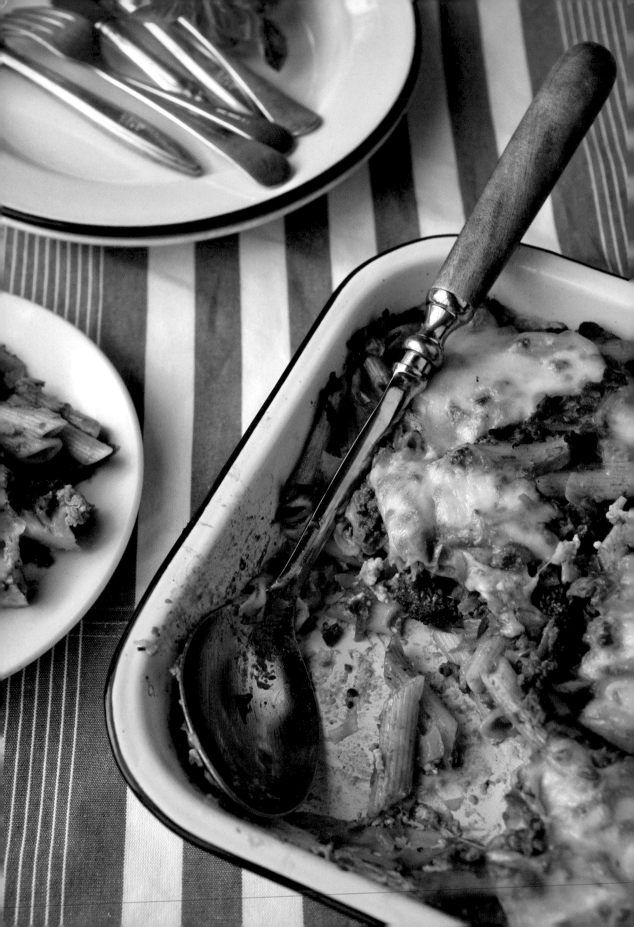

Dinner recipes

Pasta box with rainbow vegetables

This is my version of a popular Finnish family dish. I used to cook it regularly when my children were younger and had friends over as they would all enjoy it. It's a great way to get children to eat vegetables and can be prepared the day before you need it.

SERVES ❹

300 g/3 carrots
250 g/¼ cabbage
200 g broccoli
150 g/1 large onion
100 g/1 yellow pepper
100 g/1 green pepper
1 tbsp olive oil
500 g lean mince beef
800 g/2 (400 g) cans of whole peeled
  tomatoes

1 beef stock cube
4 garlic cloves, crushed
1 tsp fresh or dried basil
2 tbsp soy sauce
black and white pepper
480 g penne pasta
3 eggs
200 ml semi-skimmed milk
150 g mozzarella or grated low fat cheddar
  cheese

HOW TO PREPARE:

1 Preheat the oven to 200 ˚C.

2 Wash and peel the vegetables and chop onion.

3 Heat oil in a large non-stick pan. Fry onion until yellow and add meat. Brown gently.

4 Grate the carrots. Chop broccoli and peppers and shred cabbage.

5 Add tomatoes and the remaining vegetables to the pan.

6 Add beef stock, crushed garlic, basil, soy sauce, black and white pepper.

7 Simmer for 25 minutes, making sure you obtain a thick sauce. Do not cover.

8 Ten minutes before it is finished, add pasta to a saucepan of boiling water and cook for 10 minutes. When cooked, drain and mix together with vegetable and meat sauce.

9 Mix eggs in a bowl with milk. Lightly oil a large ovenproof dish.

10 Put the meat/vegetable/pasta mixture in the dish. Pour over the egg and milk mixture.

11 Cut mozzarella in rounds and put on top. Place in oven. Cook for 15–20 minutes until it is golden brown and melted.

APPROXIMATELY ❺❷❹ KCAL PER SERVING

Chilli con carne

I didn't invent the wheel here but this is a nice recipe.

SERVES ❹

1 tbsp olive oil
150 g/1 large onion, chopped
300 g/2 red peppers, chopped
150 g/1 yellow pepper, chopped
1 fresh chilli (or only half, depending how
   hot you want!), thinly sliced
4 garlic cloves, crushed
600 g lean minced meat

400 g/1 can chopped whole tomatoes
1 tsp herbes de Provence
1 vegetable stock cube
few drops of Worcestershire sauce
boiling water from kettle if required
800 g/8 carrots, diced
2 (400 g) cans of red kidney beans (520 g
   drained weight)

HOW TO PREPARE:

1 Heat oil in a large non-stick pan or wok. Add the chopped onion, pepper, chilli and crushed garlic. Gently fry for 2 minutes.

2 Add the minced meat, tomatoes, herbs, stock, Worcestershire sauce and boiling water from the kettle if required. Stir. Bring to the boil, then cover and reduce heat. Simmer for 15 minutes. Remove lid and simmer for another 15 minutes.

3 While chilli mixture is simmering, steam or boil the carrots for about 15 minutes or until tender.

4 Add red kidney beans to the chilli and heat thoroughly.

5 Mash the carrots with a potato masher and place in your serving dish.

6 Spoon the chilli con carne over the mashed carrots and serve.

APPROXIMATELY ❺❹❼ KCAL PER SERVING

Chicken goujons with sweet potato chips and tomato salad

How could anyone suggest I don't give nice food options!

SERVES ④

600 g chicken breasts, cut into strips
2 tbsp olive oil
2 tbsp soy sauce
1 tbsp fresh coriander/parsley, finely chopped
$^1/_2$ packet of fresh breadcrumbs
600 g sweet potatoes, peeled and cut into wedges
4 tbsp tomato ketchup

Salad
400 g/4 carrots, sliced in long strips
350 g/1 cucumber, sliced in long strips

HOW TO PREPARE:

1　Put the chicken strips in a bowl along with the olive oil, soy sauce and chopped herbs. Mix well to coat the chicken evenly and place in the fridge overnight to marinade.

2　Preheat oven to 200 ˚C.

3　Remove the bowl from the fridge and pour in the breadcrumbs. Mix well until the chicken is evenly coated.

4　Place a sheet of greaseproof paper on a baking tray and arrange the chicken on it. Place in your preheated oven and roast for 20–25 minutes depending on how thickly you have cut the strips.

5　Place the sweet potato wedges on a baking tray lined with greaseproof paper. Roast the chips in the oven for 30 minutes. The time may vary depending on your oven.

6　Prepare the salad by mixing the carrots and cucumber together.

7　Serve the chicken and chips with the salad and tomato ketchup.

APPROXIMATELY ❺❾❼ KCAL PER SERVING

Pasta carbonara à la Eva

I love pasta carbonara, but unfortunately it would set you back a week in your dietary efforts! However, this version impressed even my children, who said, 'Well done, Mum!' after trying this low calorie version. I hope you like it too.

SERVES **4**

400 g turnips
300 g wholegrain pasta
1 tbsp olive oil
1 beef stock cube dissolved in 250 ml boiling water
400 g cooked sliced ham, cut into thin cubes
4 garlic cloves, crushed
120 g low fat soft cheese
4 egg yolks
pinch of black pepper
pinch of nutmeg
parmesan, to garnish

HOW TO PREPARE:

1 Peel and slice the turnips thinly.

2 Add pasta to a saucepan of boiling water.

3 While the pasta is boiling, heat the oil in a non-stick pan and add the turnip.

4 Then add the beef stock. Cook until liquid has been absorbed.

5 Add the ham and crushed garlic. Stir.

6 Add the soft cheese and a little boiling water (50 ml) if needed to melt the cheese. Stir together.

7 After 10 minutes the pasta should be cooked. Drain pasta.

8 Add the drained pasta to the turnip, ham and cheese mixture. Blend together.

9 Add the egg yolks and stir.

10 Sprinkle with black pepper and nutmeg.

11 Grate some parmesan cheese over the cooked dish.

APPROXIMATELY **580** KCAL PER SERVING

Peppers stuffed with feta cheese and pine nuts

After this, anyone would turn vegetarian!

SERVES **4**

light spray oil
200 g easy cook rice
200 g/1 large onion
50 g peppadews
1 tbsp olive oil
400 g/1 (400 g) can of chopped tomatoes
1 tbsp tomato purée
200 g low fat feta cheese
100 g pine nuts
8 yellow peppers

tinfoil

HOW TO PREPARE:

1. Preheat oven to 200 °C.
2. Line 2 baking tins with tinfoil and spray with oil and spread out with fingers.
3. Cook rice in boiling water for 20 minutes and drain.
4. Chop the onions and peppadews.
5. Heat the oil in a large non-stick pan. Add onion, cover and sauté for a few minutes.
6. Then add tomatoes, peppadews and tomato purée to make the tomato sauce. Simmer for 5–10 minutes, uncovered so that sauce thickens.
7. Mash the feta cheese with a fork. Mix together with tomato sauce, pine nuts and rice in a bowl.
8. Slice the top off the peppers. Scrape out and discard all the seeds and white pith. Set peppers upright in the baking tin.
9. Scoop the rice and tomato mixture into the peppers. Put pepper lids back on top of the peppers.
10. Bake in the oven for 30 minutes until peppers start to wrinkle and blister.

APPROXIMATELY **540** KCAL PER SERVING

Four Seasons pizza à la Eva

This is an all-time family favourite. The secret of the low calories and healthiness is the thin base and the vegetables. Perfect for a guilt-free Saturday night in.

SERVES **4**

Pizza dough
¼ tsp salt
1 regular baking yeast sachet
200 ml lukewarm water
1 tbsp olive oil
300 g white flour

Tomato sauce
1 tsp olive oil
150 g/1 onion, chopped
400 g/1 (400 g) can of chopped whole
    tomatoes
pinch of black pepper
1 beef stock cube

Filling
230 g sweetcorn (drained weight)
200 g cooked sliced ham, chopped
400 g/4 tomatoes, sliced
100 g/1 onion, sliced thinly
125 g mozzarella cheese, grated

Salad
400 g/4 carrots, grated
juice of 1 lemon
4 tbsp balsamic vinegar

HOW TO PREPARE:

1 To prepare the pizza dough: Mix salt, yeast, water and olive oil in a bowl. Add flour slowly and mix with your hand to create a round ball. Cover the bowl with a clean tea towel and leave dough to rise in a warm place for 40 minutes.

2 To prepare the tomato sauce: Heat oil in a non-stick saucepan or a wok. Gently fry the onion first, and then add the can of tomatoes, black pepper and beef stock cube. Cover and simmer for approximately 3 minutes to create a thick sauce.

3 Preheat oven to 200 ˚C. Line a baking tray with greaseproof paper. Sprinkle the baking tray with flour.

4 Flour a table surface. Sprinkle some flour on the dough and place it on floured surface. Spread dough out with fingers.

5 Use a floured rolling pin to create a round pizza out of the dough. Use extra flour if needed when rolling. Roll the dough around the rolling pin and transfer to baking tray. Spread it out.

6 Cover pizza with the tomato sauce. Sprinkle with the sweetcorn, then the ham, tomatoes and onion, finishing with the mozzarella.

7 Put in oven for 10–15 minutes until dough is cooked and cheese melted.

8 To prepare the salad: Mix together the grated carrots and lemon juice and serve with balsamic vinegar.

9 Serve the pizza with the salad.

APPROXIMATELY 500 KCAL PER SERVING

Caprese omelette

I used to cook this at least once a week when I was studying in Italy—it's a really easy, healthy student meal. You see, I was healthy even as a student!

SERVES ❹

1 tbsp olive oil
8 eggs
375 g/3 (125 g) packets of light mozzarella cheese, grated or sliced
10 basil leaves, chopped
pinch of salt
pinch of freshly ground pepper
8 slices of wholemeal bread
4 tbsp tomato ketchup
800 g tomatoes, sliced

HOW TO PREPARE:

1 Heat the oil in a large non-stick pan, which has a lid.
2 Break the eggs into the pan and cover.
3 When eggs are almost firm, add the mozzarella cheese, basil and a pinch of salt and pepper. Cover and turn the heat down to very low. Cook for approximately 2 minutes.
4 Toast the bread and spread with ketchup.
5 When cheese is melted, divide in four and serve with sliced tomatoes and toast.

APPROXIMATELY ❺❶❶ KCAL PER SERVING

Twice-baked potatoes

This wasn't originally my idea, but I changed the ingredients and it seems to have worked out really well.

SERVES **4**

1.2 kg/4 large rooster potatoes
500 g/1 cauliflower
200 g low fat crème fraîche (less than 3 per cent fat)
1 tbsp soy sauce
pinch of ground black pepper
415 g/1 (400 g) can baked beans
1 tbsp olive oil
4 bacon rashers, chopped, with fat removed

HOW TO PREPARE:

1 Preheat oven to 200 ˚C.

2 Scrub potatoes and prick them all over with a knife. Place them on a baking tray and bake until a knife penetrates easily, 50–55 minutes.

3 While the potatoes are baking, chop the cauliflower into florets and place in a steamer. Cook until soft.

4 When potatoes are cool enough to handle, cut them in half lengthways and scoop out the pulp, leaving a thin shell.

5 Mash the potato pulp with the cauliflower, crème fraîche, soy sauce and pepper.

6 Spoon the mixture back into the potato shells. Put the potatoes back on the baking tray and bake for 10 minutes.

7 Place the baked beans in a saucepan and cook for 3 minutes.

8 Heat oil in a frying pan and add chopped rashers. Cook for approximately 2 minutes until done.

9 When potatoes are ready, serve with rashers sprinkled on top and a side dish of baked beans.

APPROXIMATELY **500** KCAL PER SERVING

CHAPTER 11

Chapter 11:
Emotional issues with food

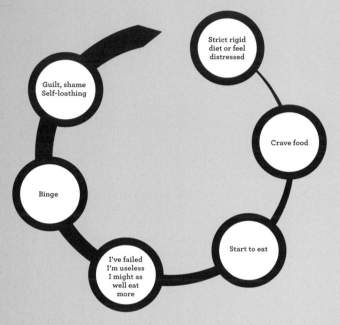

- Strict rigid diet or feel distressed
- Crave food
- Start to eat
- I've failed I'm useless I might as well eat more
- Binge
- Guilt, shame Self-loathing

ALTHOUGH FOR SOME people being overweight is merely down to lack of education and bad habits and consequently eating the wrong foods, I am aware that, for others, issues surrounding weight are deep-rooted and food is used as a coping mechanism for emotional distress. If you consider your issues to be more than a mere lack of education regarding food, then you may consider undergoing cognitive behavioural therapy at the same time as you embark on a diet. Cognitive behavioural therapy may help you to change your thoughts, beliefs and behaviours around food and help you to develop new ways of coping with your problems. This goes beyond the scope of this book.

Cognitive restructuring can help you:

- **Avoid dichotomic (black and white) thinking.**
- **Change negative thoughts.**
- **Prepare for relapses.**

Below are some techniques for changing your eating behaviour. Some of them were mentioned in Chapter 4 but it's worth examining them again. Repetition of these activities is vital so that they become part of your normal daily eating routine.

- **Establish a regular eating routine:** Eat 3 meals a day and have 2 planned snacks throughout the day.

- **Keep a food diary:** This is a very helpful tool when trying to change your eating habits. It forces you to register everything you eat and helps to stop mindless eating.

- **Control portions:** A contributory cause of excess weight and obesity is portions that are too big. You need to begin to monitor your portion size to prevent overeating. Serving your food on a smaller plate can help to reduce your portion size because the plate will not look empty.

- **Eat slowly:** It takes up to 20 minutes for your brain to register that you are full. Eating very fast means you will be inclined to overeat because you do not receive a signal from the brain to stop eating. To slow down the eating process, chew your food well and savour every bite. Put down your knife and fork between each bite. Using small knives and forks, teaspoons or chopsticks is another good way to reduce the amount of food you eat in one bite to help slow down your eating.

- **Establish a place for eating** such as the kitchen table or a specific place in your office. This will prevent grazing all day long.

- **Make sure you are aware of the food you are eating.** Avoid picking while watching TV or reading the paper. This is described as mindless eating and can lead us to overeat.

- **To help you avoid temptation, do not buy junk food.**

- **Try to get rid of 'clean your plate syndrome'.** Learn to leave a bite of food on your plate at mealtimes so that you become accustomed to not finishing everything in front of you. This will help you in your efforts to stop eating when you feel full. It is important to learn not to be obliged to eat everything that is put in front of you.

- Remember, we eat to provide our bodies with fuel to survive. Eating should not be used as a pastime. Learn to replace your continuous grazing or snacking with another activity.

Binge eating

Binge eating disorder (BED), or compulsive overeating, is characterised by periods of compulsive binge eating or overeating. There is no purging (getting rid of the food) but there may be sporadic fasts or repeated diets. Weight may vary from normal to significantly overweight.

With an eating disorder, food is not used to nourish the body. It is used to take care of emotional needs. Eating to meet psychological needs in this way is often referred to as emotional eating. Binge eating disorder is a form of emotional eating in which overeating has become a way of coping. A person with binge eating disorder becomes caught up in a vicious cycle of bingeing and dieting or restricting their food intake.

The relationship between dieting and binge eating is complex. Many people with BED report that they had episodes of bingeing before they started to diet. However, once a cycle of bingeing and dieting is established, it is the dieting that perpetuates the urge to binge.

Binge eating disorder is thought to affect up to 4 per cent of the general population.

Binge eating puts a lot of stress on the digestive processes and on the metabolism, and stomach cramps, constipation or diarrhoea can be experienced. Digestive problems such as bloating can also affect the body's capacity to absorb the nutrients it needs.

HOW TO PREVENT BINGE EATING
- Spend some time working out when you're most likely to binge—notice the thoughts that you often seem to have, the physical sensations, the emotions and how you react to them—then do something different at those times.
- Do something that takes up your attention—mindful activity.
- Compromise—eat a small portion if you really can't resist.
- Get healthier food in, rather than sugar-rich foods.
- Drink 6–8 glasses of water each day.
- Seek help—others will support you.
- Keep a food diary to assess your current intake.

- Create a simple menu plan with a suitable health professional—and stick to it! For example, 3 meals and 3 snacks per day.

- Weigh yourself no more than once a week.

- Have an exercise contract—again, agreed with a suitable health professional. Stick to it! (Guide—30 minutes of moderate exercise each day, include, e.g. getting off the bus one stop early, taking the stairs instead of the lift.)

- Use medication appropriately and only as prescribed—avoid laxatives, diet pills, diuretics.

- Eat with trusted family and friends rather than alone.

- Reward and treat yourself with something other than food when you've done well—something relaxing or fun.

- Use a Cravings Diary to record your cravings and help you to deal with these cravings so you can overcome them next time.

THINK DIFFERENTLY
- Pause, take a breath, don't react automatically.

- Try to understand the links between thoughts, feelings and behaviours.

- Practise positive self-talk—encourage yourself, tell yourself: 'I can do this, I am strong and capable'—find an affirmation that works for you (even if you don't believe it at first!) Write it down and memorise it for when you need it.

- Be aware of those unhelpful thinking habits, including 'compare and despair'—comparing yourself with others—which trigger upsetting thoughts.

- Ask yourself:
  - Is there another way of looking at this?
  - Am I getting things out of proportion?
  - Am I underestimating my ability to cope?
  - Am I mind-reading what others might be thinking?
  - Am I doing that black-and-white thinking? There are shades of grey! I don't have to be 100 per cent perfect. It's OK to be just OK.
  - What advice would I give someone else in this situation?
  - Am I putting more pressure on myself, setting up expectations of myself that are almost impossible? What would be more realistic?
  - Just because I *feel* bad doesn't mean things really *are* bad.
  - What would the consequences be of responding the way I usually do?
  - Is there another way of dealing with this? What would be the most helpful

and effective action to take (for me, for the situation, for the other person)?

- Am I exaggerating the good aspects of others, and putting myself down? Or am I exaggerating the negatives and minimising the positives?

When dealing with cravings or trying to break a binge, in addition to the information above:

- Write down what you eat whilst you binge.

- Practise relaxation techniques—try lots and find one that works for you.

- Put on some music—sing and dance along, or just listen attentively (use music that is likely to help you feel good.

- Try meditation or prayer.

- Write down your thoughts and feelings—get them out of your head.

- Just take one step at a time—don't plan too far ahead.

- Pamper yourself—do something you really enjoy, or do something relaxing.

- If you have a setback and binge—tell yourself it's OK, it's only once—don't dwell on it too much (try to see what triggered it so that you can then get back onto your self-help plan).

Coping with failure

You may have taught yourself, or your parents taught you, to comfort yourself with food. Think about a crying toddler—how often do you see parents giving their child something to eat to calm the child down.

When people are ready to change to a healthier way of living, they sometimes want it to happen in one go. They become convinced that once they have made up their minds to change, the extra weight is simply going to disappear.

How do you react when you fail? You have been good all day long but then your colleagues want to go out for dinner and you are invited. You decide to go but intend to be good. While others drink alcohol you sip on sparkling water but you slip and give in to temptation. The way you behave the following morning is what will make the difference in the long term. Don't be negative. What happened yesterday is in the past but today you will try to stick to your plan.

Yes, it is disappointing not to be always able to do what we have decided but in the end we are all human. When you feel better, the positive aspects of your weight loss slowly become more important than treating yourself.

Try to find the good habits and behaviours that you are not doing often enough. It is easier to capitalise on our good habits than start to create a totally new habit. For example, you might be in the habit of having a cup of hot water first thing in the morning but then during the day you don't drink enough. Let's try to get you having another cup of water mid-morning. You like vegetables and eat them every day for lunch but when you get home you couldn't be bothered to cook, so now we need to get you into the habit of eating them twice a day.

Chain of eating

In order to get your eating under control, you need to realise that it is not only important to control the moment of eating but what happens prior to this. Many things influence the moment of eating, creating a chain effect with many links. When the links have been identified, it is easier to break the chain. The earlier you break the chain, the easier it is to control your eating.

Chapter 12:
Phase 4—
2,000 kcal diet

PHASE 4 IS the maintenance plan and eventually you should progress to this once you have reached a healthy weight, regardless of which phase you started on. However, there are some exceptions. The calorie content of this phase may exceed the energy requirements of petite women and they should use Phase 3 as their maintenance plan. Also, although this is considered a maintenance plan, men can actually continue to lose weight in this phase as they have higher energy requirements than women. A man will lose weight at a slow rate of about 0.5 kg (1.1 lb) per week on this phase if exercise is included. For this reason, it is a suitable weight-loss plan for a man who does not have much weight to lose or who does regular strenuous exercise.

This phase is nutritionally complete and based on the 'eat well' plate to provide you with all your nutritional requirements. Again this phase is based on a breakfast, lunch and dinner with a greater choice of snacks. This is a low GI plan. In other words, it is based on foods that have a low Glycaemic Index and are broken down and released slowly in the body. This helps to keep energy levels balanced. Eating regularly and avoiding high sugar foods will ward off sugar cravings. Of course, calorie counting and portion control will still be important elements of this phase to ensure you do not exceed your 2,000 kcal/day. However, portions are larger and more food choices are included in this phase. It is important to remember that although you have lost weight, if you consistently exceed your energy requirements the weight will go back on! As I said in Chapter 1, it is a well-known fact that people put on an average of 0.5–2 kg (1.1–4.4 lb) of extra weight per year unless they actively work to maintain their weight. The same will apply to you. If you resume your old eating habits, you will resume your old shape.

Side effects

There are no side effects to this phase. It is a healthy eating plan that should not be considered a diet but a lifelong positive lifestyle change. This is how we should eat.

Alcohol

Alcohol may be included in small amounts, such as the odd glass of wine or 1–2 spirits a week on Phase 4. This can be beneficial from a social point of view and it also encourages dietary compliance from people who find it hard to follow plans that completely eliminate alcohol. However, alcohol does contain calories and if the quantities are not kept to a minimum, it may raise your total daily calorie intake significantly. Also, as alcohol lowers blood sugar levels, you may experience a craving for carbohydrates, 'the munchies'. These cravings are difficult to ignore and will jeopardise your diet success. So remember, keep alcohol to a minimum and try to save it for special occasions. Reducing alcohol has many health benefits, not only good for your waistline.

Exercise

Now that you are in the maintenance stage of your diet, exercise should play a key role in your new and improved lifestyle. It is recommended that you do 30–60 minutes of activity most days. This can be in the form of walking, swimming, running, etc. Try to incorporate exercise into your everyday life by taking the stairs instead of the lift or walking to work instead of getting the bus. Another good way to make sure exercise becomes part of your daily routine is to join a gym, a group or a team sport or take an activity class. Another option would be to adopt a rescue dog. Now you have somebody who needs and appreciates the exercise you do together. I have three dogs! You do not need to run marathons to maintain your weight but it is important to move more. Exercise burns off calories, meaning that on the days that you eat a little bit more it will be outweighed by exercising. You will find it difficult to maintain your new goal weight if you do not include exercise and you may have to be more careful with your diet. As well as helping you to maintain your weight, exercise has many other benefits. It will tone your body, make you feel happier and give you a more positive outlook on life—who wouldn't want all that?

How much energy is consumed during exercise?

The body weight is of vital importance in determining how many calories are burnt during exercise. The higher the weight, the more calories burnt—some good news for those with a higher BMI.

Here are some examples of how many calories a person will burn for different exercise levels:

One hour's exercise	Calorie consumption 70 kg (11 st)	For weight 100 kg (15st 10lb)
Slow walk 4 km/h	190 kcal	270 kcal
Brisk walk 6 km/h	330 kcal	470 kcal
Slow run speed 9 km/h	600 kcal	880 kcal
Run speed 12 km/h	850 kcal	1,200 kcal

(Source: Pertti Mustajoki, Ulla Leino, 2002, Kustannus Oy Duodelim Laihdu Pysyvästi – Hallitse Paindasi)

This is all fine but how many people weighing 100 kg can walk briskly for an hour and keep a 6 km an hour speed? People with a high BMI are unable to exercise to the point where it will make a substantial difference to their weight loss.

Tools to assist in exercise

Pedometers can be quite motivating because you can easily monitor your day-to-day activity. Pedometers also tend to increase the amount of exercise you do because as soon as you wear one, you are subconsciously more likely to increase your exercise level as you become more aware of your activity levels.

I like heart-rate monitors. I use one when I walk/run as it motivates me to start running again when my heart rate drops and I keep running until I can't any more. It's interesting to see the heart rate number and it also tells me how long I've been running. I also have a GPS running watch, but spend more time trying to figure out how it works than actually using it!

Eating out

If you continue to monitor your diet and portion sizes, the occasional meal out should not make a huge difference...within reason—so enjoy! Of course you can choose the lower calorie options on the menu, such as lean meats or fish with vegetables or salad and a moderate portion of rice or pasta, but exercising regularly and watching your diet 80 per cent of the time means you can allow yourself a little of what you fancy the odd time.

Low fat—a big fat lie

Because obesity is characterised by excessive body fat, it is commonly believed that it is partly a result of excessive fat consumption, hence a low fat diet is recommended to prevent and treat obesity. Today it seems that this concept is taken too literally and many people think that buying all low fat products is the sole answer to their weight problems. Over the past 10 years our average fat intake has decreased, but levels of excess weight carry on increasing! A question we must ask ourselves is 'Although we are eating less fat, why are we not getting thinner?'

Some low fat products are quite misleading in that they are not hugely reduced in calories, as they lead us to believe. This is because a reduction in dietary fat tends to cause a compensatory rise in carbohydrate consumption. When the fat content in a product is reduced, something needs to take its place. This 'gap' is typically filled with carbohydrates and sugar. Take a packet of 'low fat' crisps. There is 25 g of fat (per 100 g) compared with 38 g in the original version, i.e. 34 per cent less fat. However, the carbohydrates have increased from 48 g to 58 g in the low fat version and the total calorie reduction is only 12 per cent. So as you can see, often the calorie intake is only slightly reduced when compared with the original version. Although the product does have a reduced calorie content, often the taste suffers from these artificial alterations and it does not satisfy us the same way the original version did. People also tend to eat double the quantity of the low fat version because they are under the illusion that the calories are so low that this will not make a difference to their overall calorie consumption. Personally I buy very few low fat products.

I am not objecting to all low fat products as many are very good and have significantly reduced fat and calorie levels. These products can play a major role in weight reduction diets. For one thing, they allow the inclusion of low calorie alternatives to our favourite foods in our diet. This means people will not feel deprived and will have a better chance of succeeding in losing weight. In addition, the range of foods that can be included in the diet is now greatly increased.

The problem is that we have become blind with obsession and are missing the bigger picture. The low fat trend has stifled our education on the benefits of different food and a balanced diet. If we use all low fat products but continue to eat a diet rich in takeaways and junk food, we will not gain much benefit from their inclusion in the first place. Low fat products do have a place in our diet, but only if overall calorie content is controlled.

So, by attempting to reduce the fat levels, we have created a situation where our satiety levels have dropped and we end up eating more. If you follow an overall healthy diet, it is OK to include some products that are full fat, taste good and keep you satisfied. Particularly if, like me, you are maintaining your weight, the occasional use of full fat butter, cheese, milk or chocolate will make your diet more enjoyable. They will not cause weight gain if used in moderation, the rest of your diet is balanced and you lead an active lifestyle.

Meal options

Breakfast 400 kcal, Lunch 450 kcal, Dinner 800 kcal, Snacks 350 kcal

Breakfast

1 *Korvapuusti* with *café au lait*
2 *Pytti pannu* (Finnish-style healthy breakfast)
3 Banana 'ovencake'
4 Homemade oatmeal waffles with strawberry syrup

Lunch

You could alternatively make a salad, depending on the calories. See the Salad section on p.201. Or you could make a bowl of filler soup from the Soup section on p.191.

1 Rice salad, Italian style
2 Tortilla cigars
3 Green lentil feta cheese salad
4 Eggs flamenco
5 Penne all'arrabbiata
6 Vegetarian avocado couscous salad

Remember, you can also select meals from any of the previous phases.

Dinner

1 Semolina cakes
2 Creamy beef with baked potatoes
3 Cottage pie à la Eva
4 Homemade mini-burgers
5 LasagnEva
6 Sweet curry prawn sauce with egg noodles
7 Beetroot meatballs
8 Butternut chickpea red curry

Snacks

Choose 2 snacks a day (up to 350 kcal in total), preferably 1 mid-morning and 1 mid-afternoon.

1 Strawberries and crème fraîche: 100 g strawberries with 2 tbsp low fat crème fraîche (76 kcal)
2 1 whole grapefruit sliced, low calorie sweetener and 2 tbsp low fat crème fraîche (119 kcal)
3 1 medium apple or half a banana cut into pieces with 1 tbsp crunchy peanut butter on it (138 kcal)
4 Crispy apples: wash 1 small apple and chop in slices. Cover in 1 tbsp honey and roll in 10 g rice krispies (160 kcal

Top row, left to right: pytti pannu, home-made oatmeal waffles with strawberry syrup; bottom row, clockwise from far right: penne all'arrabbiata, semolina cakes, sweet curry prawn sauce with egg noodles, banana 'ovencake', beetroot meatballs

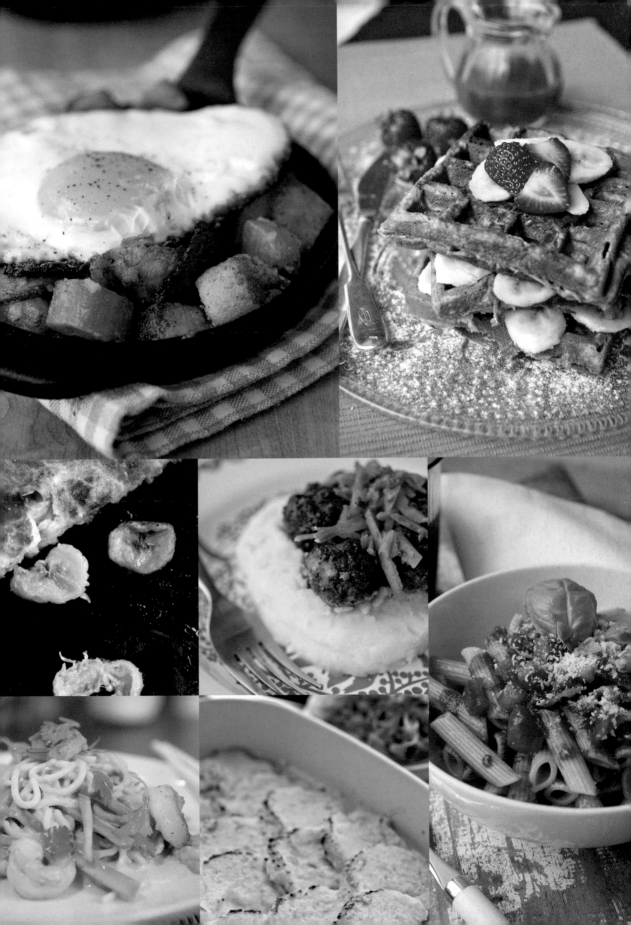

Breakfast recipes

Korvapuusti with *café au lait*

Every mother in Finland makes korvapuusti *on Saturdays and the smell of it reminds me of home baking. It's like Danish pastry but healthier.*

MAKES APPROXIMATELY **3 0**

250 ml water
250 ml low fat milk
150 g butter
2 (7 g) sachets of fast action bread yeast
200 g sugar (divided)
1 tbsp cardamom pods, ground with a
   pestle and mortar (to obtain seeds)
2 eggs
160 g oatflakes

100 g raisins
500 g wholemeal flour
250–500 g white flour
50 g 70% dark chocolate (or cocoa
   powder) (divided)
Café au lait
100 ml full cream milk
100 ml water
1 tsp coffee (or to your taste)

HOW TO PREPARE:

1 Add water and milk to a pot and heat until lukewarm. Add butter to the pot and allow to melt on a low heat while stirring continuously.

2 Put yeast and 150g sugar in a bowl and add the milk/water/butter mixture. Note that if mixture is too hot, it will kill the yeast.

3 Add the cardamom seeds and break an egg into the bowl and mix.

4 Start adding oatflakes, raisins, wholemeal and white flour and begin kneading with your hands to obtain a soft dough. Add only small amounts of flour at any time to ensure that the dough is absorbing it. The dough is ready when your hand no longer sticks to it.

5 Run hot water into the sink and place the bowl with the dough in the hot water and cover with a tea towel so that it rises. Leave covered for 30 minutes until the mixture doubles up.

6 Flour a clean surface using remaining flour.

7 Put your dough on the surface and using your hands knead it into a cylindrical shape. Cut the dough in half and cover one half with a kitchen towel.

8 Place the other dough half on a floured surface.

9 Roll it into the shape of a pizza base using a floured rolling pin. Roll the dough in one direction only.

10 When you are satisfied that the dough is evenly rolled, sprinkle 25 g sugar over the dough.

11 Grate your dark chocolate and sprinkle 25 g of it over the dough base.

12 Roll the dough over lengthways until it resembles a long thin sausage as per picture.

13 Cut the dough from one end into triangle shapes. Continue doing this until you have made 16 triangles from the dough.

14 Push your thumb into the centre of the pastry to create a circular indent.

15 Place the triangles on a baking tray lined with greaseproof paper.

16 Repeat steps 9–15 with the other dough half.

17 In a bowl crack an egg and whisk it.

18 Glaze the pastries with the egg and then place them in a preheated oven at 200 ˚C for 6–8 minutes until golden.

OPTION: You can have 2 *korvapuustis* or you can have 1 *korvapuusti* with a coffee made with 100 ml milk diluted with 100 ml water. Alternatively, if you have a coffee machine, you could make a cappuccino.

APPROXIMATELY ②⓪⓪ KCAL PER *KORVAPUUSTI* AND ⑦⓪ KCAL FOR CAFÉ AU LAIT

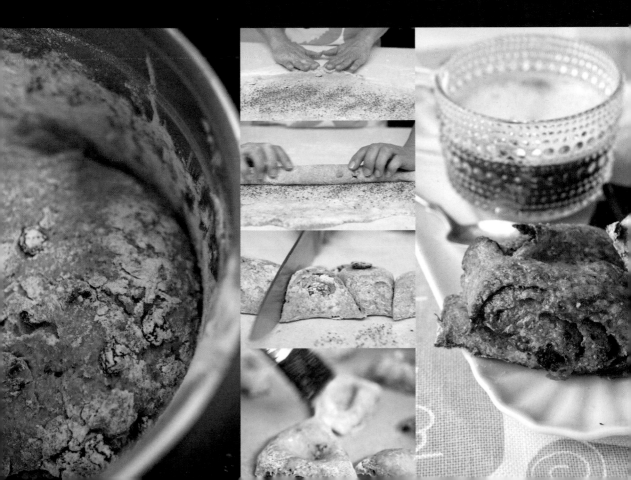

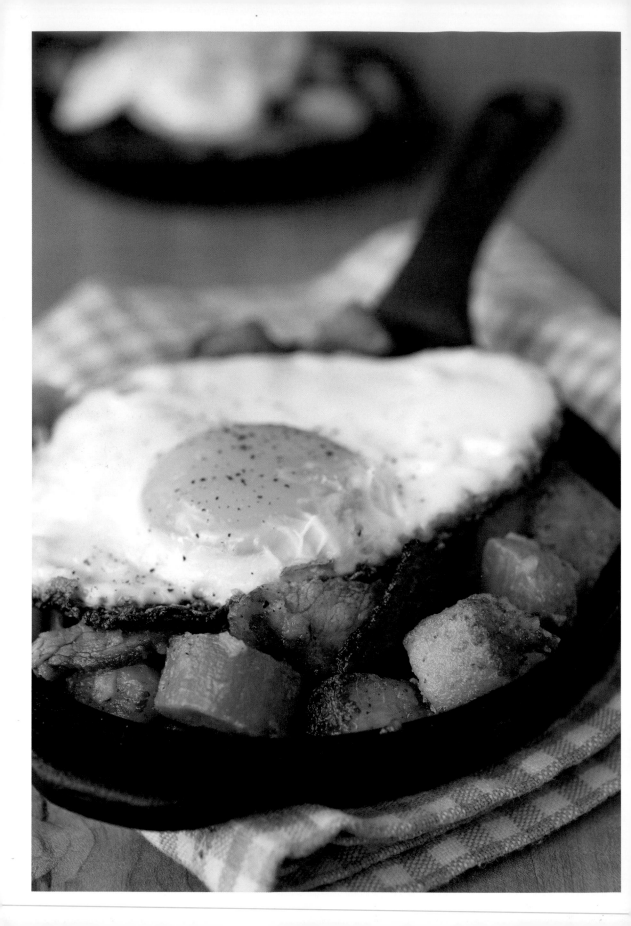

Pytti pannu (Finnish-style healthy breakfast)

This is a typical Finnish midnight snack or brunch recipe. It's healthier than it looks!

SERVES ④

500 g/4 medium organic potatoes
400 g/4 organic carrots
2 tbsp olive oil
300 g/2–3 onions
150 g organic pork rashers
4 medium eggs

HOW TO PREPARE:

1 Wash the potatoes. If using organic potatoes, there is no need to peel them as the skin is a good source of fibre. Also wash your carrots. Peel them if you are not using organic carrots. Boil for 15–30 minutes, depending on size, until al dente. Do not overcook the potatoes. (Ideally this should be done the night before preparing the breakfast.)

2 Dice your onions and fry in oil in a good non-stick pan until yellow.

3 Chop your potatoes into cubes and add to the frying pan.

4 Cut carrots into rounds. Also add these to the frying pan.

5 In the meantime, cut your rashers into cubes using kitchen scissors. Organic rashers are recommended as they are low in salt.

6 Cook these in their own fat on a good non-stick pan until crispy.

7 When rashers are crispy, add them to the potatoes, onion and carrots. Cover and cook until the vegetables are crispy.

8 Break 4 eggs into the non-stick pan in which you fried the rashers. You will not need to add oil as there should be enough fat left in the pan from the rashers. Cover and fry the eggs until they are cooked to your taste.

9 Serve the potato mixture on 4 plates and place an egg sunny side up on top. Your breakfast is now ready.

APPROXIMATELY ③⑧⓪ KCAL PER SERVING

Banana 'ovencake'

I often make this easy recipe on Sunday morning for my sons before they play rugby. It's a brilliant combination of protein and carbohydrates (1 banana = 25 g carbohydrates!).

SERVES ④

Batter
30 g Dr Eva's healthy spread (see p.207)
180 g/2 medium bananas (weighed unpeeled)
250 g/4 medium eggs
500 ml low fat milk
350 g flour
1 tbsp natural unrefined cane sugar (optional as bananas are quite sweet on their own)
Sauce
1 lemon
1 medium banana

HOW TO PREPARE:

1 Preheat oven to 200 °C.

2 Put spread on an oven tray and allow to melt.

3 Peel and chop bananas in circles and place them on the baking tray.

4 Place in oven for 3 minutes to allow to fry.

5 In the meantime, break eggs into a bowl and whisk.

6 Add the milk, gradually whisking together with the eggs all the time.

7 Add the flour and sugar and whisk all together until you obtain a smooth mixture.

8 Leave the mixture to stand for 30 minutes if you have the time, or you could make the mixture the night before.

9 Remove the bananas from the oven. Lift the tray and allow the melted spread to disperse evenly.

10 Pour the pancake mixture evenly over the bananas and place in the oven for 20 minutes.

11 To make the sauce, squeeze 1 lemon to obtain juice.

12 Peel and chop a banana and liquidise in a jug with the lemon juice to obtain a zesty sauce for your pancake.

APPROXIMATELY ❸❾❻ KCAL PER SERVING

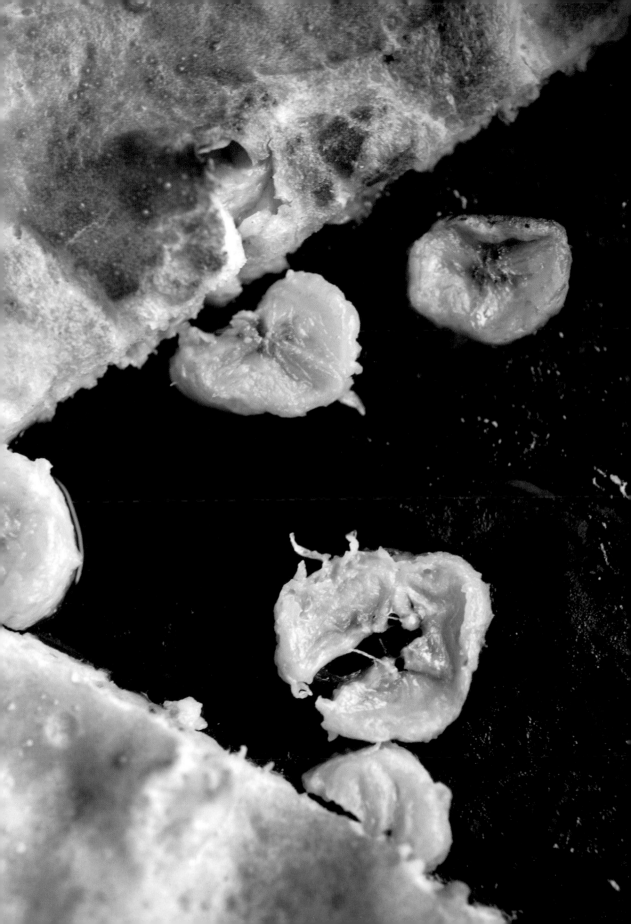

Homemade oatmeal waffles with strawberry syrup

Eating this, you really don't think you are on a maintenance diet. It just shows how you can make healthy food that is super tasty.

SERVES ❹

Wet ingredients
1 medium egg
150 ml milk
1 tbsp honey
1 tbsp groundnut oil
¼ tsp vanilla extract
80 g/1 banana peeled weight

Dry ingredients
110 g white flour
50 g wholegrain rolled oats (porridge oats)

½ tsp ground cinnamon
½ tsp bicarbonate of soda
½ tsp baking soda

Syrup
3 tbsp water
3 tbsp low calorie sweetener
200–300 g strawberries

light spray oil
waffle maker

HOW TO PREPARE:

1 Crack an egg into a bowl and whisk together with milk, honey, oil, vanilla extract.

2 Peel and mash the banana and blend together with the egg/milk mixture. You may need to use a hand blender.

3 In a separate bowl mix the flour, oats, baking soda, cinnamon and bicarbonate of soda.

4 Slowly add the wet mixture to the dry ingredients, blending them all the time. Do this until you have created a smooth mixture.

5 Heat the waffle maker to a medium heat (I use a Cuisinart waffle maker level 3) and spray some light spray oil on it.

6 Pour the waffle mixture into the centre of the grid and spread it out evenly until it completely covers the lower grid. Close down the lid and allow to cook. Leave for about 4 minutes (or until your machine beeps to indicate it's ready).

7 In the meantime, wash some strawberries and chop into small pieces. Add to a pot with the low calorie sweetener and the water.

8 Place on a medium heat and stir continuously until the strawberries melt and the juice creates a syrup.

9 When the waffles are ready, serve on a plate and top with the strawberry syrup.

NOTE: Although this is quite a bit of work for 4 waffles, it is better to make this recipe in small quantities as the waffles taste best when they are warm and fresh.

APPROXIMATELY ❷❾❿ KCAL PER SERVING

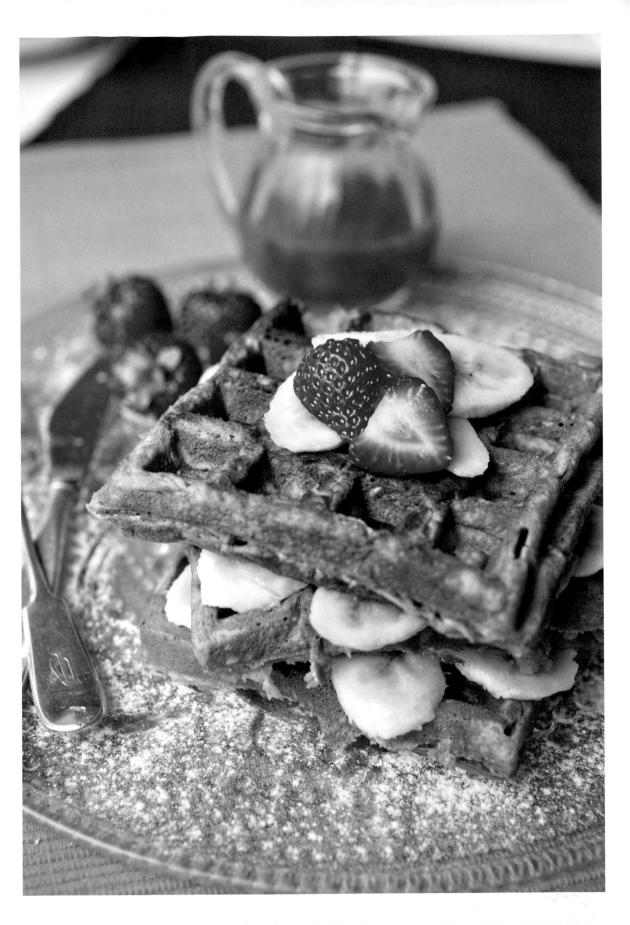

Lunch recipes

Rice salad, Italian style

You find this in every restaurant in Italy. This version just has more vegetables.

SERVES ❹

1 litre water
pinch of salt
200 g easy-cook long-grain rice
1 green apple
1 red apple
2 Frankfurter sausages
8 gherkins, drained

50 g/1 small red onion
200 g/2 carrots, peeled
200 g low fat cheese (less than 30
  per cent fat)
Dressing
8 tbsp low fat vinaigrette or
  balsamic vinegar

HOW TO PREPARE:

1 Add a pinch of salt to 1 litre of water and boil. Add rice, simmer for 20 minutes and
   then drain.

2 Remove cores from green and red apples and cut into very small cubes.

3 Cut the sausages, gherkins, onion and carrots very small.

4 Cut the low fat cheese into very small cubes.

5 Mix rice and all other ingredients in a bowl.

6 Serve with salad dressing.

APPROXIMATELY ❹❺❺ KCAL PER SERVING

Tortilla cigars

This is a quick way to make wraps. But bought versions usually have high calorie fillings.

1 tbsp soy sauce
1 tbsp oyster sauce
600 g chicken, cut in strips
1 tbsp olive oil
2 garlic cloves, crushed
100 g baby sweetcorn
100 g French beans
100 g sugar snap peas
light spray oil
600 g Chinese cabbage leaves, cut in thin strips
black pepper, to taste
6 wholewheat tortillas
2 tbsp sweet chilli sauce (optional)
400 g/4 vine tomatoes, sliced
juice of 1 lime

HOW TO PREPARE:

1 Mix soy sauce, oyster sauce and chicken strips in a bowl.

2 Heat a large non-stick pan. Add oil, garlic and chicken.

3 Add sweetcorn, French beans and sugar snap peas. Cook for 7–8 minutes until chicken is cooked.

4 In separate wok or large pan, heat some spray oil and add the Chinese cabbage and black pepper. Cook for 2–4 minutes.

5 Heat the tortillas in a microwave or preheated conventional oven for 1 minute.

6 Place a tortilla on a serving plate and cut in half. Fill with the cabbage and chicken mixture. Fold to create a cone shape.

7 Drizzle with sweet chilli sauce.

8 Mix the tomato slices with the lime juice.

9 Serve 3 tortilla cones per person with the tomatoes.

APPROXIMATELY ❹❶❼ KCAL PER SERVING

Green lentil feta cheese salad

I like feta cheese—it's a great source of protein for vegetarians, who typically don't get enough in their diet.

SERVES ❹

1 litre water
1 bay leaf
50 ml vinegar
400 g canned green lentils
400 g crisp heart lettuce
200 g light feta cheese
150 g/1 red onion (raw)
600 g/4 large tomatoes
12 slices of bacon (optional)
Salad dressing
1 tbsp balsamic vinegar
60 ml/½ pot low fat natural yoghurt

HOW TO PREPARE:

1 Boil green lentils in 1 litre of water in which you put 1 bay leaf and 50 ml of vinegar. It will take approximately 25 minutes. Drain and leave to cool down.

2 Wash, dry and shred the lettuce and place on your plate. Add cooled green lentils.

3 Break the feta cheese with a fork and sprinkle over the lentils.

4 Peel and chop the onion in thin slices and place over the lentils.

5 Wash the tomatoes and cut in thin slices.

6 If you choose to add bacon, grill until crispy and add to salad.

7 Prepare the dressing by mixing balsamic vinegar with half a pot of natural yoghurt and drizzle over salad.

APPROXIMATELY ❸❻❸ KCAL PER SERVING

Eggs flamenco

I love eggs and I love spicy food so this is a combination of two of my favourite things. It's also quick and easy to make.

SERVES **4**

150 g/1 onion
150 g/1 green pepper
150 g/1 red pepper
1 tbsp olive oil
2 garlic cloves, crushed
1 tsp fresh ginger, grated
1 tsp ground cumin
1 tsp ground coriander
½ tsp red chilli powder
½ tsp turmeric
1 vegetable stock cube
8 plum tomatoes, chopped
2 tbsp white wine vinegar
8 large eggs
wholemeal bread, toasted (no more than 50 g per head)

HOW TO PREPARE:

1 Peel and chop the onion and peppers.
2 Heat the oil in a large non-stick pan.
3 Add onion, peppers, garlic and ginger.
4 Stir in herbs and spices, stock cube and tomatoes.
5 Close lid, simmer for 15 minutes.
6 Add vinegar.
7 Make 8 hollows with the back of a spoon.
8 Crack an egg into each hollow.
9 Cover and cook until eggs are done to your liking, 2-4 minutes.
10 Serve with toasted wholemeal bread.

APPROXIMATELY **340** KCAL PER SERVING

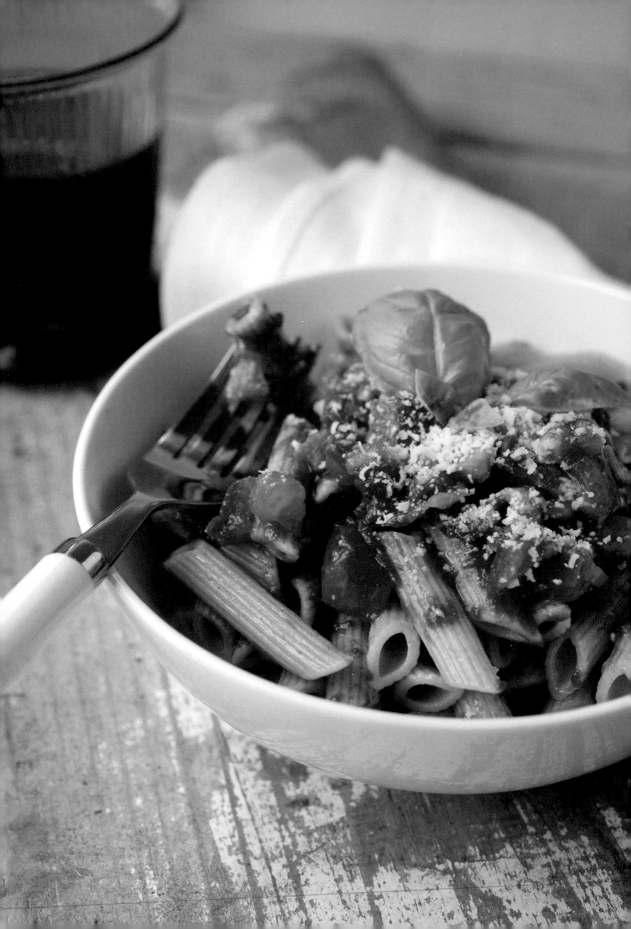

Penne all'arrabbiata

This is a typical Italian dish and it's so easy.

75–100g/½–1 onion
250 g fresh plum tomatoes (or 200 g/½ (400 g) can tomatoes)
75 g wholewheat penne pasta
1 tsp olive oil
1 tsp chopped chilli
30 g parmesan cheese

HOW TO PREPARE:

1 Put water on to boil for your pasta.

2 Peel and chop onion.

3 Wash plum tomatoes and cut in quarters.

4 Cook pasta as per instructions.

5 Heat a teaspoon of oil in a non-stick pan and fry onion.

6 Add chilli and plum tomatoes to pan. Cover with a lid to allow moisture to escape from tomatoes. Every now and then remove the lid and break the tomatoes with a spatula.

7 Remove the lid from the pan when liquid has formed to allow some of the liquid to evaporate and a sauce to form.

8 Drain pasta when cooked. Add your sauce and top with grated parmesan cheese.

APPROXIMATELY ❹❺❶ KCAL PER SERVING

Vegetarian avocado couscous salad

Although they contain 'good' fats, avocados are high in calories.

SERVES ❹

140 g couscous
300 g cherry tomatoes or 3 whole tomatoes
200 g green beans
100 g/1 red onion
70 g lamb's lettuce
100 g cashew nuts
1 avocado
Salad dressing
2 garlic cloves
1 small chilli
15 ml olive oil
100 ml coriander
3 tbsp Diet 7up
1 tsp grated lemon peel

HOW TO PREPARE:

1 Prepare your couscous as per the instructions.

2 Chop tomatoes finely and toss through couscous.

3 Steam the green beans and chop onion finely. Mix all through the couscous.

4 Serve on a bed of lamb's lettuce.

5 Top with couscous mixture and cashew nuts.

6 Then make your salad dressing. Peel and crush garlic cloves. Deseed a chilli and chop finely. Mix in a bowl with olive oil, coriander, Diet 7up and lemon peel. Drizzle over your salad.

7 Cut an avocado down the centre and remove the stone. Cut the avocado in quarters and serve a quarter with each salad portion.

APPROXIMATELY ❹❽❿ KCAL PER SERVING

Semolina cakes

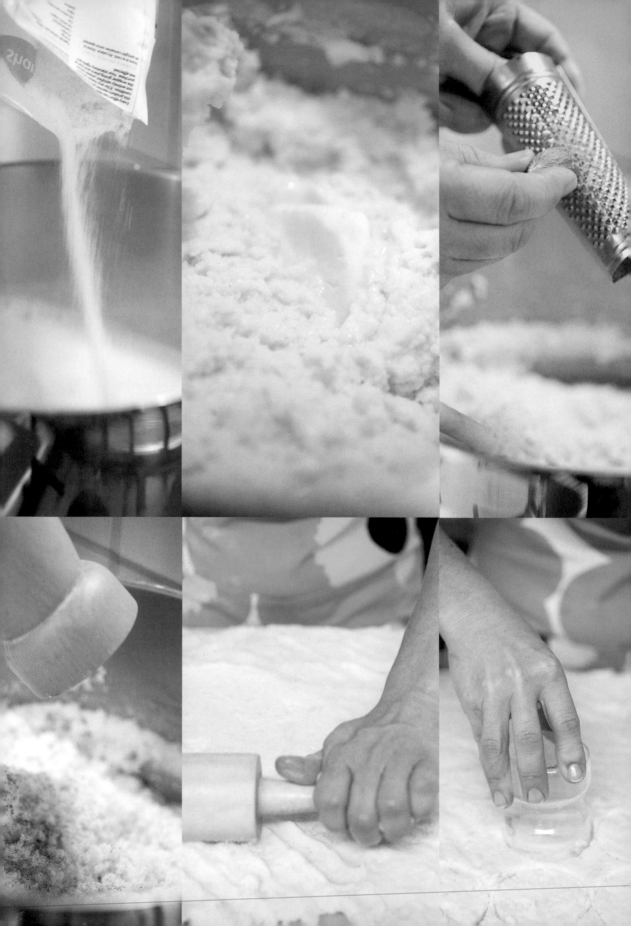

Dinner recipes

Semolina cakes

This is a classic Italian recipe. Good things come to those who wait—I promised you carbs and butter would be re-introduced once you reached the maintenance phase so here you go! Hard to believe you can make such a delicious dish out of simple ingredients.

SERVES ❹

1.9 litres milk
500 g semolina flour
2 tbsp butter
5 egg yolks
pinch of salt
pinch of black pepper
pinch of nutmeg
300 g parmesan cheese, finely grated
400 g carrots, grated
juice of 1 lemon

HOW TO PREPARE:

1   Heat the milk in a big pot and add the semolina flour, mixing continuously to avoid lumps. Add the butter, egg yolks, salt, black pepper and nutmeg.

2   When the mixture forms a sort of dough, remove the pot from the heat and spread out mixture over a clean kitchen surface with a rolling pin, or with the help of a kitchen spoon.

3   Put water in a dish to wet the top of a glass. Wet a glass and use it as a stencil to create round flat cakes. Put the cakes in an oiled oven dish. When you have filled your dish, sprinkle cakes with parmesan cheese.

4   Serve with grated carrot drizzled with lemon juice.

APPROXIMATELY ❻❺❿ KCAL PER SERVING

Creamy beef with baked potatoes

Most of the fibre in old potatoes is in the skin. Wash it well so you can eat the whole thing.

SERVES **4**

800 g–1 kg/4 rooster potatoes
2 tbsp olive/rapeseed oil
450 g/3 onions
400 g ready cut beef strips
1 tbsp grated ginger
1 tsp hot chilli paste (optional)
2 tbsp soy sauce
2 tbsp black bean sauce
200 ml half fat crème fraîche
400 g/4 carrots
juice of 1 lemon

HOW TO PREPARE:

1 Preheat oven to 200 ˚C.

2 Wash the potatoes and pierce them with a fork. Place in the oven.

3 Heat the pan and add the oil.

4 Cut the onion in half moons and add to frying pan. Leave to cook for 4–5 minutes.

5 Add the beef to the frying pan and allow to cook for 5–8 minutes.

6 Add the ginger, chilli paste, soy sauce and black bean sauce and stir continuously.

7 When the food is almost cooked, add the carton of crème fraîche. Cover the pan and allow to simmer for approximately 5 minutes.

8 Cut the ends off the carrots and peel them. Grate the carrots.

9 Serve the creamy baked potatoes with grated carrot drizzled with lemon juice and beef.

APPROXIMATELY **500** KCAL PER SERVING

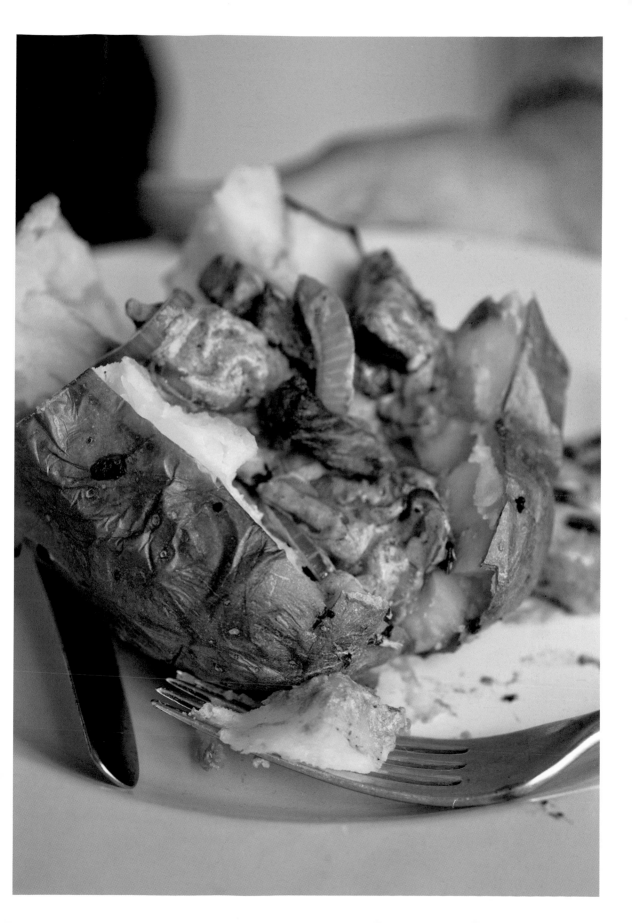

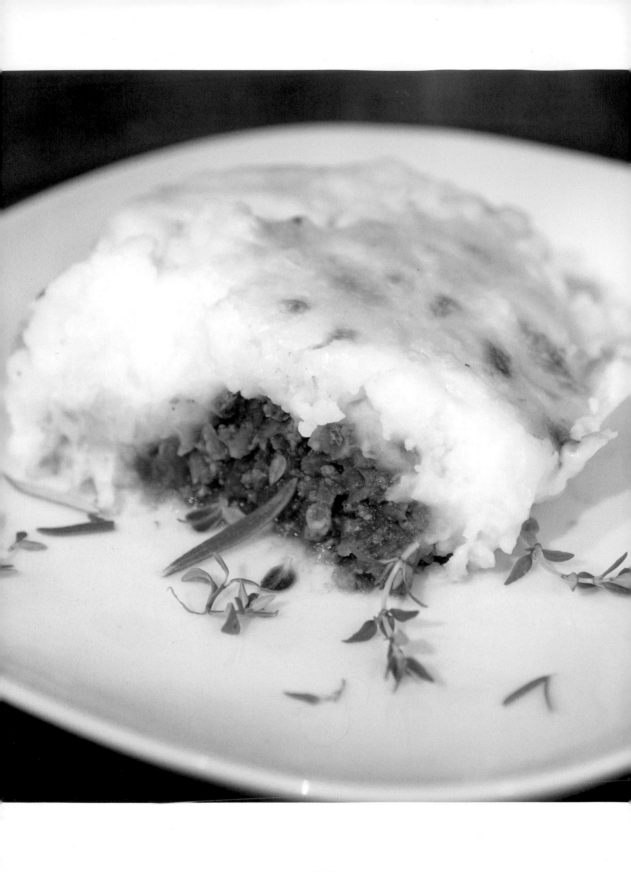

Cottage pie à la Eva

I love oven casseroles. The secret here is the large amount of vegetables mixed with the minced meat.

SERVES ❹

200 g/1 onion
600 g/4 potatoes
400 g/4 carrots
1 tbsp olive oil
4 garlic cloves, crushed (optional)
500 g minced meat (lamb or beef)
800 g/2 (400 g) cans of whole peeled tomatoes
freshly ground black pepper
1 vegetable or beef stock cube dissolved in 250 ml boiling water from kettle
100 ml low fat milk
light spray oil
100 g low fat cheddar cheese, grated

HOW TO PREPARE:

1 Peel and chop the onion and potatoes. Grate the carrots.

2 Heat the oil in a pan. Add the onions and garlic and fry for 1-2 minutes.

3 Add mince and cook on high heat, stirring all the time until browned.

4 Add the carrots, tomatoes, pepper and stock. Bring to the boil and cook for about 30 minutes until it forms a thick sauce.

5 In the meantime, place potatoes in the pot and cover with boiling water. Simmer for 15 minutes until potatoes are soft. Then drain off water and mash potatoes with the low fat milk.

6 Use the spray oil to cover the inside of an oven dish and spread out with fingers.

7 Pour the sauce into oven dish and then spread mashed potatoes over it.

8 Sprinkle grated cheese on top and place in oven at 200 ˚C for 25 minutes.

APPROXIMATELY ❹❼❸ KCAL PER SERVING

Homemade mini-burgers

Now I'm giving too many tasty fast-food options!

SERVES **4**

6 oval wholemeal pittabreads, cut in half
Burgers
1 tbsp olive oil
400 g/4 courgettes, grated
150 g/1 onion, chopped finely
600 g premium minced meat
2 eggs
3 tbsp soy sauce
pinch of black pepper
Sauce
400 ml low fat natural yoghurt
1 tbsp wholegrain mustard
1 tbsp medium curry powder
1 tsp ketchup (optional)
Side salad
3 butter head lettuces, washed and the leaves separated
200 g/2 cucumbers, diced
400 g/4 tomatoes, diced

HOW TO PREPARE:

1 Heat oil in a wok or non-stick pan, add the courgette and onion. Cook until moisture evaporates, approximately 5 minutes.

2 Mix the cooked courgette/onion with the minced meat and the eggs in a bowl. Add the soy sauce and pepper.

3 Form little mini-burgers and return to your pan on a medium heat. Cover and leave until fully cooked and browned. (Halfway during cooking turn the burgers so that they cook evenly on both sides.)

4 If you feel the burgers are sticking, add a little hot water to the pan.

5 While the burgers are cooking, make your sauce by combining the yoghurt, mustard and curry powder in a bowl. (You can add a teaspoon of ketchup, if you like.)

6 In each pitta pocket, place some lettuce, cucumber, tomato and 1 burger and spoon over sauce.

7 Use the rest of the lettuce, cucumber and tomatoes to make a side salad.

APPROXIMATELY **680** KCAL PER SERVING

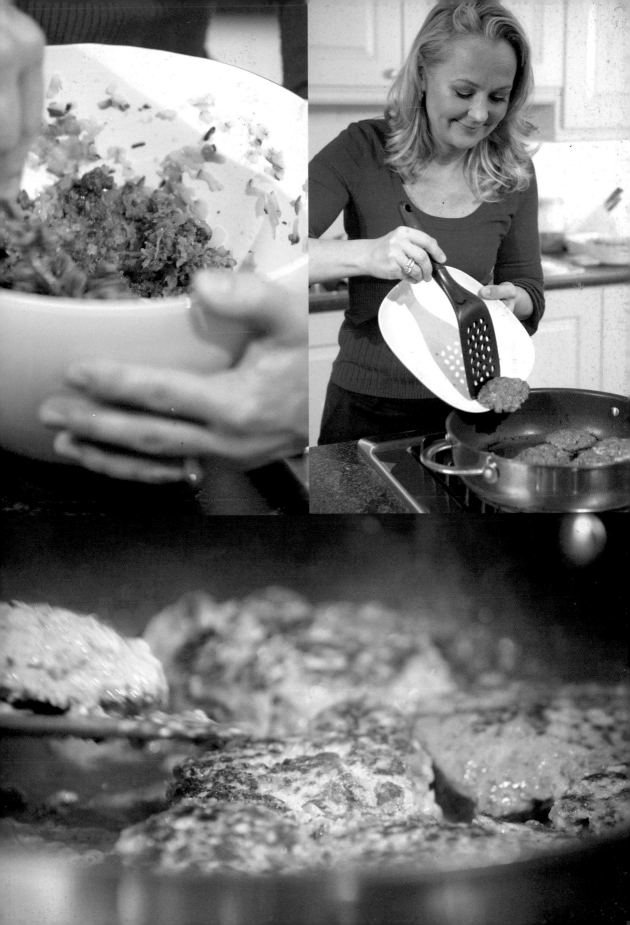

LasagnEva

That's not a spelling mistake! I'd like to think I'm getting better every day at making these low calorie versions.

SERVES ❹

Bolognaise sauce
150 g/1 onion
125 g/1 red pepper
125 g/1 yellow pepper
300 g/3 courgettes
300 g/3 carrots
1 tbsp olive oil
400 g minced meat
800 g/2 (400 g) cans of whole peeled
   tomatoes
1 beef or vegetable stock cube or 1 tbsp
   Swiss vegetable vegan bouillon
black pepper (freshly ground if possible)
4 garlic cloves, crushed

1 tbsp tomato purée
pinch of paprika
1 tsp oregano
White sauce
20 g butter
2 tbsp flour
800 ml semi-skimmed milk

light spray oil
200 g/10–11 (Barilla) lasagne sheets
200 g low fat feta cheese

tinfoil
deep rectangular oven dish 30 cm × 27 cm
   × 6 cm

HOW TO PREPARE:

1 Chop the onions and peppers. Grate the courgettes and carrots.

2 Heat the oil in a large non-stick pan. Add mince and onions.

3 When mince is browned, add the carrots, courgettes, peppers and tomatoes. Stir.

4 Add stock cube, black pepper, garlic, tomato purée, paprika and oregano. Cover and let it simmer for 35–45 minutes, stirring occasionally.

5 Prepare white sauce. Melt the butter in a pan. Add the flour and milk. This sauce is meant to be very liquid and only minimum quantity of butter and flour is used to keep the calorie content down. You need this sauce only to moisturise the lasagne sheets.

6 Use spray of oil to coat oven dish and spread out with fingers. Pour the white sauce in the bottom so that the lasagne sheets are covered. Add a layer of mince/vegetable mixture and over that another layer of white sauce and on top of that another lasagne sheet. Carry on with white sauce and mince/vegetable mixture for another layer or two so that the last layer is mince/vegetable mixture. Crumble the feta cheese over the top.

7 Cover with tinfoil and place in oven at 200 °C for approximately 30 minutes.

APPROXIMATELY ❼❷❻ KCAL PER SERVING

Sweet curry prawn sauce with egg noodles

This is incredibly quick and easy to prepare. Very nice!

SERVES ④

1 tbsp olive oil
150 g/1 onion, cut in half rings
400 g/4 carrots, cut in very thin strips
1 vegetable stock cube dissolved in 100 ml of boiling water from the kettle
3 tbsp soy sauce
1 tbsp medium curry powder
1 tbsp low calorie sweetener
150 g low fat soft cheese
200 ml low fat milk
600 g large cooked and peeled king prawns
300 g pre-cooked ready to wok Thai-style ribbon noodles
pinch of coriander or parsley, to garnish

HOW TO PREPARE:

1 Heat oil in non-stick pan and add onions and carrot strips.

2 Add vegetable stock, cover and leave to simmer for 10 minutes.

2 When onions and carrots are soft, add soy sauce, curry powder and low calorie sweetener. Cook for 1 minute.

3 Add soft cheese and milk and stir to create a sauce. Cover for 1 minute and then add the king prawns.

4 Add pre-cooked noodles to the wok and stir. Cover for 1–2 minutes to warm the noodles up. If you have fresh coriander or parsley, add some for extra colour and taste!

APPROXIMATELY ❺❼⓿ KCAL PER SERVING

Beetroot meatballs

This is a typical Finnish recipe, Lindström steak. *It is usually cooked on a cast-iron pan with lots of butter but oven cooking it reduces the amount of butter required. These meatballs are gorgeous as finger food at children's parties and a great way of introducing vegetables into your and your children's diet.*

SERVES ❹

150 g/1–2 onions
1 tbsp olive oil
500 g minced meat
300 g/2–3 beetroot in vinegar (depending on the size), grated
3 eggs
1 tbsp soy sauce
white or black pepper
400 g/4 carrots
juice of 1 lemon
1 kg potatoes
100 ml skimmed milk
20 g butter
pinch of salt

HOW TO PREPARE:

1 Preheat oven to 200 ˚C.
2 Chop the onion and fry in the olive oil until yellow.
3 Mix the minced meat, onions, beetroot and eggs in a big bowl.
4 Add the soy sauce and pepper.
5 When you have a nice smooth texture, use a teaspoon or ice-cream scoop to mould approximately 25–30 balls.
6 Place the meatballs on a baking tray lined with greaseproof paper.
7 Cook for 20 minutes, depending on your oven.
8 In the meantime, grate the carrots and add the juice of a lemon.
9 Peel potatoes and cut in cubes. Boil until soft. Drain the water and mash with skimmed milk and butter. Add a pinch of salt.
10 Serve the meatballs with carrot and mash.

APPROXIMATELY ❻❶❶ KCAL PER SERVING

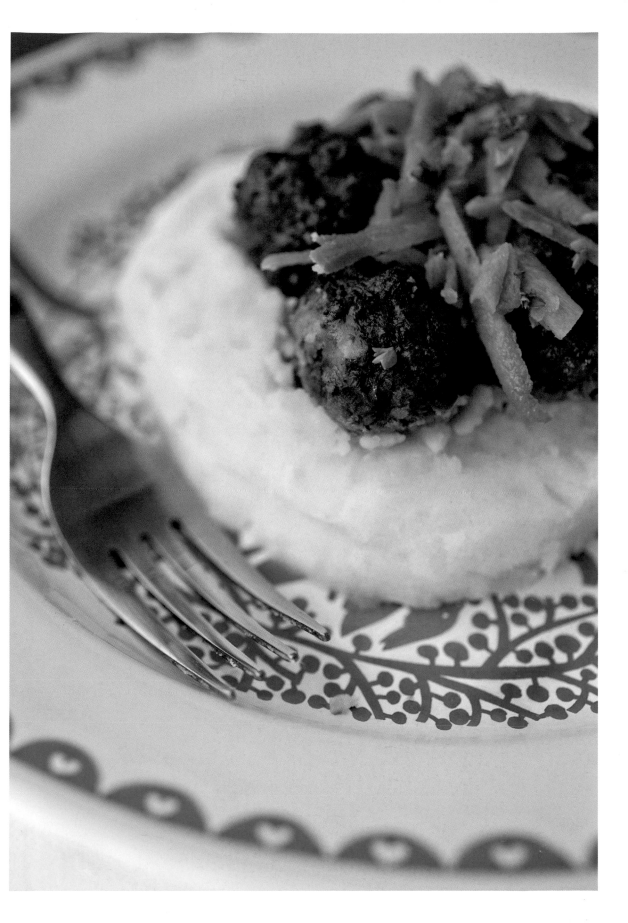

Butternut chickpea red curry

This is a delicious vegetarian option. If I could come up with more recipes like this, I would become a vegetarian!

SERVES 4

200 g wholemeal rice
600 g butternut squash
1 tbsp olive oil
500 g baby onions (peeled but not chopped)
5–15 ml/1–3 tsp Thai red curry paste (depends on how spicy you like it)
1–2 tbsp ginger
2–3 pieces galangal

250 ml boiling water
2 tbsp fish sauce
2 tbsp soy sauce
3 garlic cloves, crushed
1 tsp turmeric
400 g/1 can chickpeas (drained)
400 ml/1 can of light coconut milk
fresh coriander leaves, to serve

HOW TO PREPARE:

1   Cook rice according to instructions.
2   Peel and chop the butternut squash into medium-sized cubes.
3   Heat the olive oil in a large non-stick pan.
4   Add the baby onions first and fry for 3 minutes until brown.
5   Then add red curry paste, ginger and galangal and stir.
6   Add the butternut squash and boiling water.
7   Add fish sauce, soy sauce, garlic and turmeric and stir.
8   Cover, reduce heat and simmer for 15 minutes.
9   Add the chickpeas and coconut milk.
10 Heat for a few minutes.
11 Drain rice.
12 Serve curry with rice and fresh coriander leaves.

APPROXIMATELY 650 KCAL PER SERVING

CHAPTER 13:
Soups, salads and spreads

BY NOW YOU will be aware that I am a big fan of vegetables and believe that they form a major part of the diet of anyone who is trying to eat healthily. You always need to have a bowl of vegetable filler soup in the fridge—you can have it first thing when you walk in after a hard day's work so you're not tempted to indulge in something unhealthy. A soup will last up to three days in the fridge but you should keep a variety so you don't get tired of particular vegetables. You could cook in bulk and freeze in smaller portions. Well done—you're so organised.

Because soups are low in calories it is important to include them on Phase 1 to keep you full with minimum calories.

Note that these recipes are for more than 1 serving and so can be made in batches and frozen in individual portions for convenience.

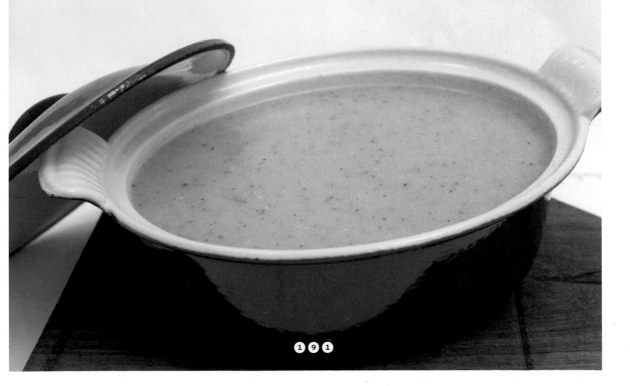

Celeriac and apple soup

800 g/1 average celeriac (pre-peeled)
200 g celery
1 small onion
2 litres water (divided)
1 vegetable stock cube
4 garlic cloves
pinch of black pepper
1 tsp grated ginger
2 bay leaves
300 g/3 cooking apples (pre-peeled)
200 ml half fat sour cream

HOW TO PREPARE:

1   Chop your peeled celeriac finely.
2   Chop celery finely.
3   Peel onion and dice it into small cubes.
4   Put both of the above ingredients into a pot with a small amount of water (approximately 500 ml) and allow to simmer on a medium heat for 5 minutes.
5   Melt vegetable stock cube in 1.5 litres of boiling water and add to pot.
6   Peel and crush the garlic and add to pot.
7   Sprinkle in black pepper.
8   Add in ginger and bay leaves.
9   Allow ingredients to simmer.
10 Then peel apple and chop finely (exclude the apple core) and add to pot after 5–10 minutes.
11 Allow to cook until all of the vegetables are soft (approximately 25 minutes in total).
12 Remove bay leaves and then liquidise the soup.
13 Allow soup to cool slightly and then add in 200 ml low fat sour cream. Mix thoroughly.

APPROXIMATELY 300 ML—**59** KCAL

Fennel and orange soup

SERVES ④-⑥

150 g/1 leek
1 garlic clove
1 tbsp olive oil
600 g/2 fennel bulbs

2 tsp grated orange peel
1 chicken stock cube melted in 700 ml
  boiling water from kettle

HOW TO PREPARE:

1 Wash and cut the leek and garlic and fry in olive oil in a wok for 5–10 minutes.

2 Cut the fennel in thin slices and add to the wok. Simmer until golden.

3 Add orange peel and chicken stock and cook for 30 minutes.

4 Liquidise with a hand mixer or in a liquidiser.

APPROXIMATELY ⑤⓪ KCAL PER SERVING

Hot mushroom soup

SERVES ④-⑥

300 g/2 leeks
200 g/1 courgette
800 g mushrooms
1 tbsp olive oil
1 tbsp instant hot and sour tom yum paste

1 litre boiling water from kettle
1 bay leaf
2 tbsp soy sauce
1 chicken or vegetable stock cube

HOW TO PREPARE:

1 Wash and chop all the vegetables.

2 Pour the olive oil into the wok and add the leeks and the hot and sour tom yum paste. Stir a few times, allowing the paste to heat to activate the flavours.

4 Start adding the sliced mushrooms and courgette. Stir a few times and add boiling water from the kettle.

5 Add 1 bay leaf, soy sauce and 1 stock cube.

6 Add hot water until you cover the vegetables and let simmer.

7 Cook for 15 minutes but do not overcook as you will destroy all the vitamins.

8 Remove the bay leaf before serving.

APPROXIMATELY ⑤⓪ KCAL PER SERVING

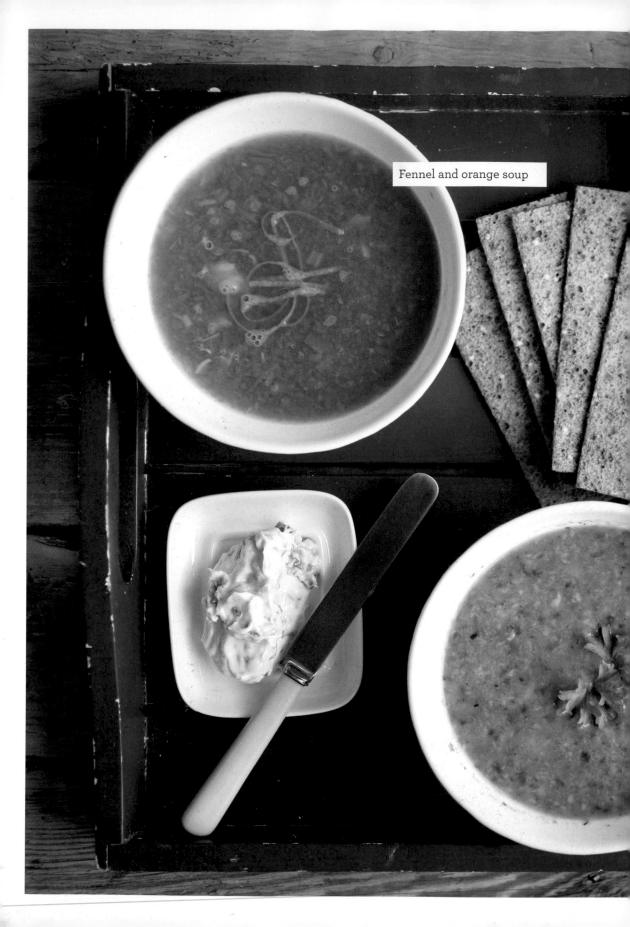

Fennel and orange soup

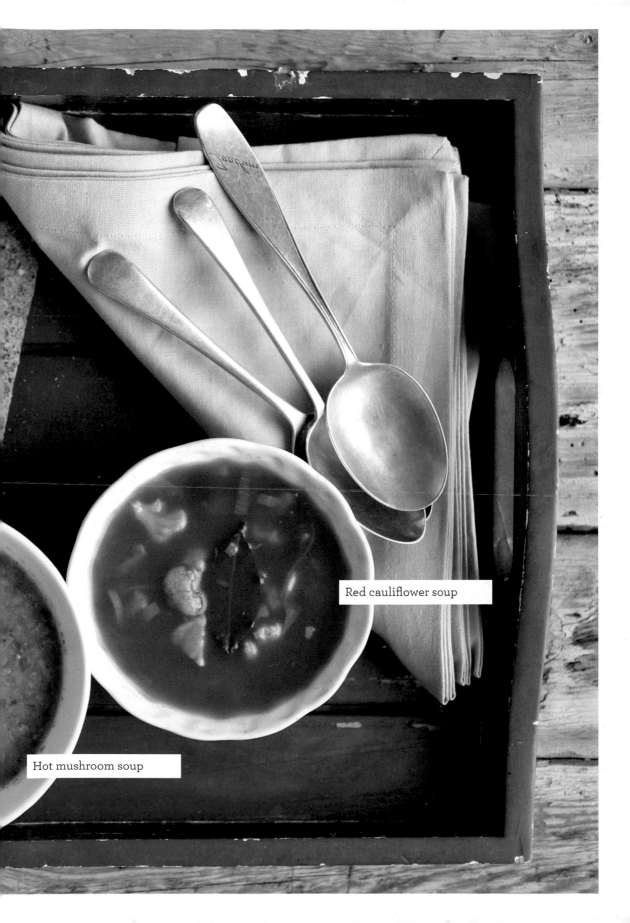

Red cauliflower soup

Hot mushroom soup

Red cauliflower soup

SERVES ❹-❻

300 g/2 leeks
700 g/1 head of cauliflower
2 tsp olive oil
½ tsp tom yum paste or other red curry paste
400 g/1 (400 g) can whole peeled plum tomatoes
½ vegetable stock cube
2 litres boiling water from the kettle
2 tbsp soy sauce
1 bay leaf

HOW TO PREPARE:

1 Wash and chop leeks and cauliflower.

2 Heat the olive oil in a wok or large non-stick saucepan.

3 Add the curry paste and allow to heat for a few minutes to activate the flavours. Then add the tomatoes to provide some moisture.

4 Add leeks and cauliflower to the wok.

5 Dissolve vegetable stock in 2 litres of boiling water from the kettle and add to the wok.

6 Add the soy sauce and bay leaf and let simmer for 20 minutes.

7 Remove the bay leaf before serving.

8 Liquidise if you prefer.

APPROXIMATELY ❺❶ KCAL PER SERVING

Hot fennel cauliflower soup

SERVES ❹-❻

600 g/2 fennel bulbs, chopped
250 g/1 big leek or 2 small ones
1 tbsp olive oil
1 beef stock cube melted in 1 litre boiling water from kettle
600 g/1 cauliflower, chopped
1 tsp turmeric
1 tsp medium curry powder
1 stick of cinnamon

HOW TO PREPARE:

1 Slightly fry the sliced fennel and leek in olive oil in a big pot or in a wok.

2 Add half of the beef stock and then add the chopped cauliflower.

3 Add the spices and the remaining stock.

4 Let simmer for approximately 20 minutes and when vegetables are soft, purée with a hand mixer or put it through a food processor for a creamy soup. Alternatively, serve as it is if you like it chunky.

APPROXIMATELY **5 0** KCAL PER SERVING

Mixed vegetable soup

SERVES **6**-**8**

150 g/1 leek
200 g/2 courgettes
60 g mushrooms
150 g/2 sticks of celery
100 g cabbage
1 tbsp olive oil
200 g cauliflower
200 g broccoli
1 vegetable stock cube dissolved in 1 litre boiling water from kettle
2 bay leaves
2 tbsp soy sauce

HOW TO PREPARE:

1 Wash the leek and cut it first lengthways in half and then in half-rounds. Cut the courgettes, mushrooms and celery into slices. Cut the cabbage in thin shreds and cut cauliflower and broccoli into florets.

2 Add 1 tablespoon of oil to a wok or pot. When oil is hot, add vegetables starting with cabbage. Stir frequently. After a few minutes add leeks, courgettes, mushrooms, broccoli and cauliflower.

3 When vegetables start sticking to the pot or wok, add vegetable stock (melted in hot water). Then add the bay leaves and soy sauce and leave to simmer for 20 minutes.

4 Remove bay leaves before serving.

5 If you prefer a creamier consistency. liquidise with a hand blender at the end of cooking.

APPROXIMATELY **5 0** KCAL PER SERVING

Spicy cauliflower soup

SERVES ④-⑥

1 tbsp olive oil
1 tsp Thai red curry paste
150 g/1 leek
750 g cauliflower

1 vegetable stock cube
1 litre boiling water from the kettle
1 tbsp soy sauce
1 tsp turmeric

HOW TO PREPARE:

1 Pour the olive oil into a hot wok or pot.

2 Add 1 teaspoon of red curry paste or less if you prefer less spicy soup. Allow to heat for a few minutes to activate the flavours.

3 Wash and chop leeks and cauliflower. Add to pot.

4 Melt the vegetable stock in boiling water from the kettle and add to the wok.

5 Add the soy sauce and turmeric and let simmer for 20 minutes. If you prefer a creamier consistency, liquidise with a hand blender at the end of cooking.

APPROXIMATELY ⑤⓪ KCAL PER BOWL

Mild cinnamon cauliflower soup

SERVES ①⓪

1 tbsp olive or rapeseed oil
1 kg turnip, cut in small cubes
2 litres boiling water from kettle
600 g/1 cauliflower, chopped in small pieces

1 star aniseed
1 cinnamon stick, broken in big pieces (so that you can remove them easily at the end!)
1 tbsp Swiss vegetable vegan bouillon

HOW TO PREPARE:

1 Place oil in a big pot and add turnip cubes. Fry for a few seconds and then add boiling water.

2 Add cauliflower, star aniseed, cinnamon stick and vegetable bouillon.

3 Let simmer until turnip is soft, approximately 30–45 minutes (depending on how big you cut turnip cubes).

4 When cooked, remove star aniseed and cinnamon stick and liquidise with a hand blender.

APPROXIMATELY ⑤⓪ KCAL PER SERVING

Spinach soup

150 g/1 leek
500 g spinach
30 g Dr Eva's healthy spread (see p.207)
3 tbsp flour

1 litre low fat milk
1 vegetable stock cube
500 ml boiling water from kettle

HOW TO PREPARE:

1 Wash and cut leeks down the centre and then in half-rounds.

2 Melt healthy spread in a pot and add leeks. Fry leeks for approximately 5 minutes.

3 Add flour and stir well until it absorbs the spread to obtain a smooth mixture.

4 Gradually begin to add low fat milk, stirring continuously to obtain a smooth sauce.

5 Dissolve stock cube in 500 ml of boiling water from the kettle. Add to the pot and stir well.

6 Wash spinach and shred in small pieces. Add to the pot and allow to cook in milky sauce. Allow to simmer for approximately 10–15 minutes and then liquidise.

APPROXIMATELY ❺❶ KCAL PER SERVING

Broccoli soup

400 g broccoli, chopped in florets
350 g cauliflower, chopped in florets
200 g/4 celery sticks, sliced
150 g/1 leek, sliced thinly
100 g/1 courgette, sliced

2 tbsp soy sauce
1 vegetable stock cube
1 litre boiling water from kettle
1–2 garlic cloves (according to taste)
pinch of white or black pepper

HOW TO PREPARE:

1 Place all vegetables in a large saucepan. Add soy sauce and stock cube dissolved in 1 litre of boiling water from kettle.

2 Add garlic and a pinch of white or black pepper or according to taste.

3 Bring to the boil. Then simmer approximately 20 minutes until vegetables are soft.

4 Liquidise if preferred.

APPROXIMATELY ⑤⓪ KCAL PER SERVING

Green curry turnip soup

SERVES ⑥-⑧

600 g/1 turnip
350 g/3 courgettes
250 g/2 leeks
200 g/½ head of celery
1 red chilli, deseeded
1 tbsp olive oil
3 garlic cloves, crushed
1 tbsp Chinese five spice

2 tbsp fish sauce
1 tbsp green curry paste
1 vegetable stock cube
1–1.5 litres boiling water from kettle
    (depending how thick you would like
    the soup)
100 ml light coconut milk

HOW TO PREPARE:

1 Wash and chop the vegetables.

2 Heat oil in a wok or large non-stick saucepan. Fry chopped turnip, courgettes, leeks and celery for a few minutes. Add garlic, spice, fish sauce and curry paste.

3 Dissolve stock cube in boiling water from the kettle. Add to pan.

4 Simmer for 30–40 minutes until vegetables are soft.

5 Add coconut milk when done.

6 Liquidise if preferred.

APPROXIMATELY ⑦⓪ KCAL PER SERVING

Salads

A salad is a fantastically easy and versatile dish, great to eat as a main course with cooked vegetables, as a side salad or in a wrap. Often the problem when people make salads is that 'lightweight' salad ingredients are used. Although these ingredients are low in calories, they are also generally low in fibre and so the salad does not have sufficient ingredients to provide long-lasting satiety. These low calorie salads are then laced with high calorie salad dressings that often contain more calories than the salad itself. Therefore the salad overall does not provide much benefit to a dieter. Here are the basic steps to prepare a satisfying, nutritious and interesting salad.

1 **BASE OF THE SALAD: This should consist of lettuce leaves. Use a variety of types to make it interesting, e.g. iceberg lettuce, crispy butter lettuce, crispy romaine lettuce, roxy lettuce, little gem lettuce, Chinese cabbage, etc. These leaves should not be too strong in flavour because they are the base of the salad. Remember, lettuce is quite low in fibre so does not contribute much to the overall fibre intake.**

2 **FLAVOUR: This can be added by using rocket leaves, spinach leaves or lamb's lettuce. They will intensify the flavour of the salad.**

3 **FIBRE: Include high fibre vegetables either raw or slightly steamed, e.g. cauliflower, broccoli, fennel, celery, asparagus, French green beans, tomatoes, white or red cabbage, pak choi lettuce or brussels sprouts. You can also use grilled vegetables such as peppers and mushrooms.**

FROM PHASE 2 ONWARDS

Taste can be added using raw onion (white and red) or spring onions, peppadews, olives, capers, leeks, gherkins, beetroot and carrots (grated or cut in julienne), etc. This group of ingredients will add extra flavour to make your salad unique.

Another popular ingredient for salads is sweetcorn. However, sweetcorn is quite high in calories (16 kcal/tablespoon) so should be used only in small amounts.

Protein

Always make sure you have a source of protein. This is where you get your longer-lasting satiety.

A typical protein serving suitable for all phases at lunchtime is approximately 100 kcal. Examples of this are:

- **50 g/1 large egg**
- **85 g/small tin tuna in brine**
- **70 g smoked or cooked salmon (98 kcal and 17 g protein) or 80 g/small tin sardines or 120 g mackerel**
- **50 g low fat feta cheese/halloumi/mozzarella/goat's cheese/2–3 slices of low fat soft cheese**
- **2–3 slices of extra lean ham/chicken/turkey**

BEANS AND LENTILS (UNSUITABLE FOR PHASE 1)
These are a great source of protein, especially for vegetarians or vegans. They are also a good source of fibre. However, they do contain carbohydrate and so should NOT be included in Phase 1. They are high in calories so portion control is important. WHO recommends a daily amount of 30 g of pulses, nuts and seeds to guard against heart disease and certain types of cancers.

A typical serving with approximately 100 kcal is:

- **100 g/⅓ can drained chickpeas (cooked from can)**
- **120 g whole drained lentils (cooked from can)**
- **125 g red kidney beans (cooked from can)**
- **30 g cashew nuts**

Carbohydrate (phases 2–4 only)

To turn your salad into a meal, include one of the following (approximately 100 kcal):

- **5 Finn Crisp crackers/3 Ryvita/5 Ryvita crackerbreads**
- **½ large or 1 small wrap/1 wholegrain pitta bread**
- **1 medium potato**
- **30 g wholegrain rice or pasta (uncooked)**
- **30 g quinoa (uncooked)**

Beetroot salad

This is my favourite salad. The scarlet colour of beetroot is thought to be a combination of the naturally occurring yellow (betacyanin) and purple (betaxanthin) pigments. These vibrant pigments are potent phytochemicals and antioxidants that work to protect damage to body cells from free radicals.

600 g/4 beetroot (raw)
600 g/4 green apples
200 g/4 celery sticks (optional)
Dressing
2 tbsp olive oil

4 tbsp orange juice
2 tbsp balsamic vinegar

grater

HOW TO PREPARE:

1   Peel beetroot and place in a bowl of water (while preparing the apples). Note that you may want to use gloves or put oil on your hands before handling the beetroot to prevent it staining your skin.

2   Peel apples.

3   Using a grater or, if you have a special grating machine, grate the beetroot and apples very fine.

4   Mix grated beetroot and grated apples together.

5   Wash and chop celery and mix with salad.

6   In a bowl, mix olive oil, orange juice and balsamic vinegar.

7   Drizzle dressing over salad and mix well.

NOTE: Salad dressing will preserve salad for 2–3 days. This recipe will serve 4 if used alone or serves 8 as part of another salad or vegetable dish. Do not be alarmed if your urine turns reddish.

APPROXIMATELY **170** KCAL PER 330 G SERVING

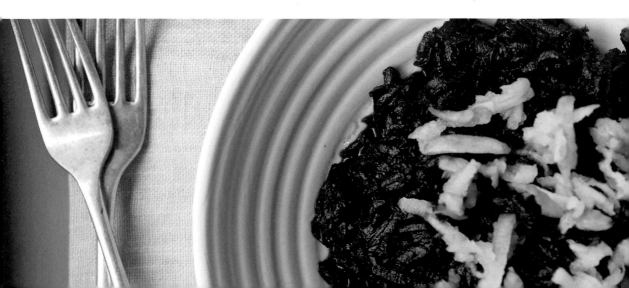

Homemade coleslaw

500 g/½ Savoy cabbage
300 g/2–3 carrots
120 g/2–3 small red onions
300 ml low fat natural yoghurt
2 tbsp readymade horseradish sauce
100 ml apple juice

grater

HOW TO PREPARE:

1 Wash and thinly peel the carrots and remove both ends.

2 Remove outer leaves of cabbage and wash the individual leaves.

3 Shred the cabbage, carrots and onions.

4 Mix together natural yoghurt, horseradish sauce and apple juice in a bowl.

5 Add the yoghurt mixture to the vegetables and mix well.

NOTE: You could make this on a Sunday and then use it during the week for your salads.

APPROXIMATELY ❶❸❺ KCAL PER SERVING

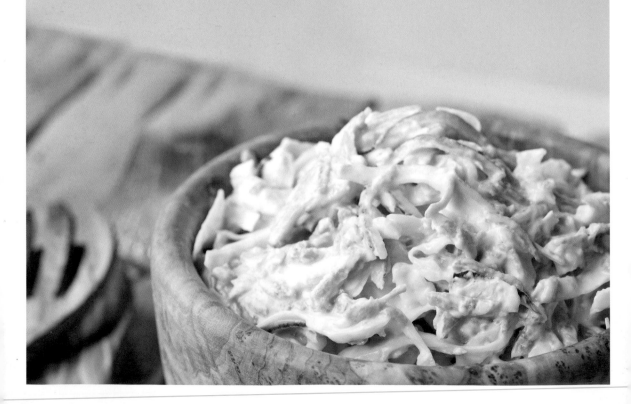

Salad dressings

SALAD DRESSINGS SUITABLE FOR ALL PHASES

French dressing: 1 tbsp balsamic vinegar, 1 tbsp lemon juice, 1 tsp mustard, 1 tbsp olive oil, salt and pepper to taste. Mix all together.

APPROXIMATELY **42** KCAL PER TABLESPOON, 0.1 G CARBOHYDRATE

Fresh fruity dressing: 3 cloves crushed garlic, 2 cm ginger, 2 tbsp fish sauce, 2 tsp low calorie sweetener, 1 tsp Thai red curry paste, juice of 1 lime, 2 tbsp orange juice. Mix all together.

APPROXIMATELY **8** KCAL PER TABLESPOON, 1.6 G CARBOHYDRATE

Creamy mint salad dressing: 350 g chopped cucumber, 10 chopped mint leaves, 20 g/3 cloves crushed garlic, 200 ml natural yoghurt, pinch of salt. Mix all together.

APPROXIMATELY **4** KCAL PER TABLESPOON, 0.6 G CARBOHYDRATE

Blue cheese dressing: 30 g Roquefort blue cheese, 100 g low fat natural yoghurt. Crumble the cheese and mix with the yoghurt. Can be used on burgers or pittas or as a dip for raw vegetables.

APPROXIMATELY **20** KCAL PER TABLESPOON, 0.9G CARBOHYDRATE

Blueberry dressing: 150 g blueberries, 100 ml orange juice, 50 ml vinegar, 10 ml mustard. Mix all together.

APPROXIMATELY **5** KCAL PER TABLESPOON, 0.8 G CARBOHYDRATE

Lemon dressing: 5 ml grated peel of lemon, 2 crushed garlic cloves, 1 small deseeded chilli, 15 ml olive oil and 3 tbsp Diet 7up. Mix all together.

APPROXIMATELY **32** KCAL PER TABLESPOON, 0.2G CARBOHYDRATE

Green pea wasabi spread

480 g frozen garden peas
4–6 mint leaves
1 tbsp tahini (sesame-seed paste)
2 tbsp low fat crème fraîche
1 tbsp ready-made horseradish sauce
juice of 1 lime
2 garlic cloves
$1/4$ tsp wasabi ready-made paste in tube or powder—
depending how much 'bite' you prefer

HOW TO PREPARE:

1 Cook peas in boiling water for 3 minutes; drain and rinse with cold water.
2 Place peas and the rest of the ingredients in a food processor or use hand blender, and process until smooth.
3 Spoon pea mixture into a serving bowl and serve with rye cracker bread or use as a dip with a crudité platter.

NOTE: If you find the taste too strong with the wasabi or any of the other ingredients, you can try using less next time!

APPROXIMATELY 15 KCAL PER TABLESPOON

Creamy egg spread

3 eggs
100 g low fat sour cream
100 g/1 shallot

HOW TO PREPARE:

1 Hard boil 3 eggs. Peel and break with a fork into a bowl. Mix together with low fat sour cream (128 kcal/100 g).
2 Chop 1 shallot finely.
3 Mix all together.

APPROXIMATELY 26 KCAL PER TABLESPOON

Dr Eva's healthy spread

100 g butter (preferably organic)
100 ml olive oil
100 ml water
2–4 tbsp parsley according to preference, or another herb, e.g. basil

HOW TO PREPARE:
1 Mix the butter with the olive oil and blend with the water. Add
  parsley (or another herb you prefer—better to leave the herbs out
  if you are using this spread for cooking). You could also add
  garlic if you wish.

APPROXIMATELY 1,700 KCAL IN 300 ML OR 85 KCAL PER
TABLESPOON

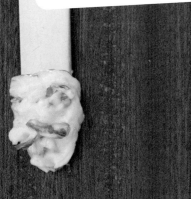

Comparison of Dr Eva's healthy spread with butter

Nutrient/100 g	Butter	Dr Eva's spread
Calories	724	419
Protein	0.4 g	0.9 g
Carbohydrate	0.3 g	0.8 g
Fat	80	45.9
Saturated	52.8	16.6
Monounsaturated	21	23.5
Polyunsaturated	2.8	2.8

Green lentil hummus spread

You will get approximately 750 g of hummus. If you want, you can make smaller portions by dividing the recipe by 4.

SERVES 4
200 g chickpeas (dry) or 400 g drained weight from can
1 tbsp + ¼ tsp baking soda
100 g green lentils (dry weight)
100 ml natural low fat yogurt
1–3 garlic cloves
1 tsp cumin
pinch of grated nutmeg
juice of ½–1 lemon
pinch of salt
1 tbsp readymade pesto
basil or mint
paprika to garnish

HOW TO PREPARE:
1 Weigh chickpeas and lentils. Discard any that are damaged.
2 Wash the chickpeas and lentils several times until water is transparent. Soak them in water with the tablespoon of baking soda and leave overnight or 5–10 hours. Then wash again. The grains should absorb the water and almost double in volume.
3 After washing them well, put them in a large pot. Cover with water and add the rest of the baking soda. Cook for approximately 20–30 minutes until the grains are soft and very easily mashed when pressed between two fingers.
4 In a separate pot boil the green lentils for 20–30 minutes until they are soft. Drain and set aside to cool down.
5 Put the chilled chickpeas in the food processor together with the cooked lentils.
6 Add the natural yoghurt and the rest of the ingredients and keep liquidising with the food processor or hand mixer until you get the desired texture. If the hummus is too thick, add some of the cooking water.
7 Serve with some chopped basil or mint and sprinkle with ground paprika spice for extra colour.

APPROXIMATELY 35 KCAL PER TABLESPOON

Dr Eva's low calorie sangria

Congratulations! You've made it to the end. Have some sangria and celebrate!

750 ml Cabernet
   Sauvignon
100 ml Jamaican rum
200 ml orange juice
200 ml ginger wine
2 tsp artificial sweetener
3 cinnamon sticks

1 litre Diet 7up
1 litre low calorie/sugar
   free lemon bitter
1 lemon, chopped
1 orange, chopped
1 lime, chopped
4 mandarins, chopped

HOW TO PREPARE:
1 Mix ingredients in a big bowl and serve with plenty of ice.

NOTE: This sangria is only 'low' in calories if served in small quantities.

APPROXIMATELY 43 KCAL PER 100 ML

Afterword

Having completed your weight-loss journey, I hope you are beginning to reap the benefits. Your energy levels should be way up, mood improved and you should generally be feeling more positive about life. At this stage you should have an established regular eating routine. This means eating three main meals with small snacks in between.

Although you will have hopefully achieved your goal weight, it is still important to monitor your eating habits as this is when bad eating habits can creep back in. Weight maintenance in itself is the biggest challenge. Aim to weigh yourself once a week to keep an eye on your weight. Remember that the changes you have made have been lifestyle changes. As soon as you revert back to your old ways of eating, you will revert back to your old shape because at the end of the day, when you eat extra calories, they have to go somewhere! Write down a list of the benefits you have gained since changing your eating habits, such as looking better, being more positive about life, having more energy and improved health. The list is endless and different for everybody but you can be sure that the benefits of maintaining a healthy lifestyle will far outweigh the benefits of returning to your old eating habits. If your old eating habits had benefited you, you would not have tried to change them in the first place. It is worth remembering this as we can often forget.

I do not wish to encourage a cycle of yo-yo dieting and I am a huge advocate of healthy living so let this be the last time you ever struggle with your weight. It's all about attitude towards food. Food should be seen primarily as the 'fuel' you need to survive, but it can be tasty and enjoyable. I hope my recipes and food essentials have given you the knowledge to make great, tasty homemade meals.

I hope you have enjoyed your weight-loss journey and have found this book helpful. I wish you every success in the future!

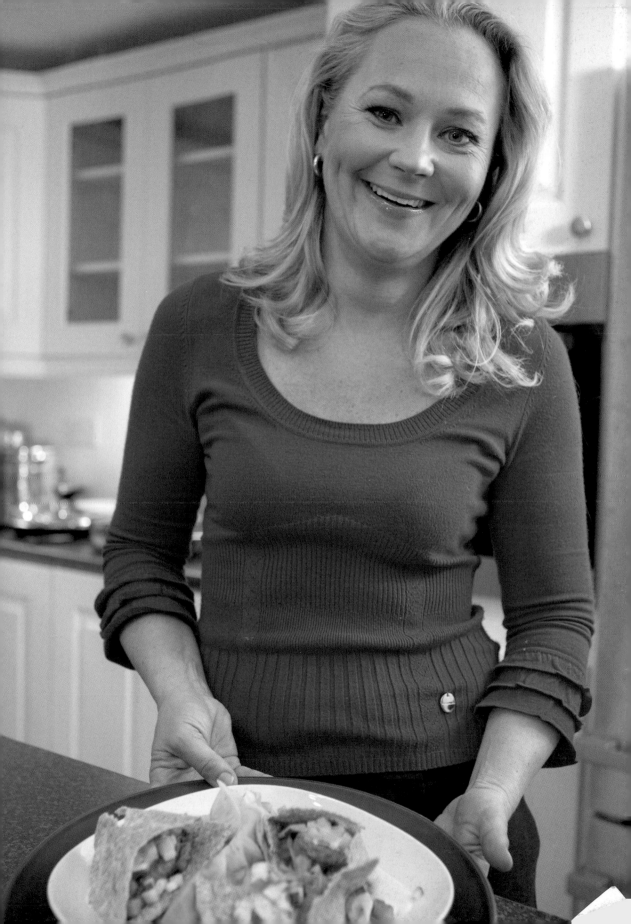

Index

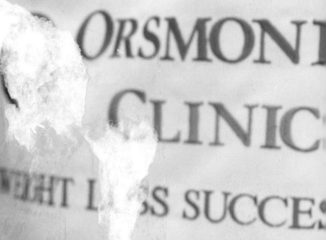

ORSMOND
CLINIC
WEIGHT LOSS SUCCES